Voice of Experience:

Stories about Health Care and the Elderly

D1502835

Samuel Brody MD
Jane K. Brody RN PhD

Publisher's Note

This publication contains the ideas and opinions of its authors. It is sold with the understanding that the authors are not providing personal or professional services (including but not limited to medical, health, legal, or financial services.) Readers are encouraged to consult competent health care providers for their care. The authors and publishers specifically disclaim all responsibility for any liability or loss incurred from the application of any contents of this book. All the case studies are fictionalized composite stories from the authors' experience and do not refer to any particular patients or their families.

Photographs by Jane K. Brody

Materials on the elderly and driving from the Family Caregiver Alliance printed with their expressed permission.

A Prayer for Healing written by Rabbi Marc Gruber printed with his expressed permission

ISBN   978-0-5781-2630-2

Printed in the United States of America

This book is dedicated to our parents:

Charles and Ethel Brody
Sumner and Betty Kreplick

They were true role models of integrity, caring, and compassion

And to our siblings who shared the joys and sorrows and also contributed greatly to our parents' care

We also dedicate this book to our patients and their families for allowing us to be part of their lives.

Table of Contents

Section Three: Quality of Life

Section Four: Health Care Decision Making

Section Five: Beyond the Stories— Thoughts to Consider

Acknowledgements

Thanks to our friends and colleagues who gave support and encouragement along the way. Jane's sister, Dr. Sandra Fernbach, Mr. Don Milner, and Dr. David Thickman, helped with the editing. Rabbi Marc Gruber provided wonderful insights about our book.

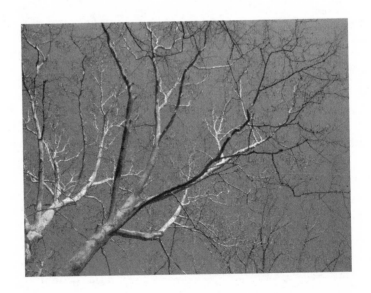

Foreword: Voice of Experience: Stories About Health Care and the Elderly

We have been married for 40 years and have been health care providers—Jane, a nurse and Sam, a physician—for almost as long. We often share our professional experiences with each other to help deal with our feelings and to think through the extraordinary events which are part of our work. Our experiences with the declining health and deaths of our parents have also added a personal dimension to our continued exploration of how to provide the best health care for people as they age.

We will try to impart some of the knowledge we have gained from family experiences, the patients and their families whom we treat, the residents and students that we teach, and family and friends who seek our council. This book is another way to share what we have learned and have been taught through our interactions within the health care system. The stories reflect actual events but have been modified to maintain privacy and to help present the ideas we wish to communicate to the reader more clearly. Some stories will be composites of several experiences. We have written them in a conversational rather than a scholarly tone. We want to sound as if we were talking to you personally. We hope that each of you will find a story or two that resonates with you and addresses an issue of your concern.

Throughout this book we use terms like the older adult or the elderly interchangeably. These terms along with others such as "the aged" and senior citizens do not specifically or accurately define an age category. The AARP (formerly known as the American Association of Retired Persons) accepts members after the age of fifty. Social Security has a variety of ages for retirement beginning at 62 years. We hear that 60 is the new 50 and 70 is the new 60. This reflects advances in the health of the general population and a change in societal attitudes. Jane remembers the grandmother of her youth with white hair, no makeup, plain dark dresses, rolled down stockings and sensible shoes. She was shocked when much later in life she realized that the picture in her mind reflected the period when her grandmother was only in her early sixties—the age we are now. The older adult, we will say, is 60 to the early 80's. The old old is 85 plus in years. By percentages, the old old is the age group that is the fastest growing segment of the population.

In this book use pseudonyms for the people in our stories. Sometimes we use the first names and sometimes we use the more formal title and last name. We recognize the need to address all patients by the names they prefer. Some want the respect of a more formal approach; others like the intimacy implied by the use of first names. The choice of name is reflective of the situation also. With Sam knowing people over long periods of time, the use of first names is understandable. (Many choose to call him Sam rather than Dr. Brody) When Jane is in the hospital working with people for the first time, the use of title and last name is more appropriate.

Although we will refer to financial issues when discussing the stories, we do not offer much specific guidance. The system is too complex and ever changing for us to provide detailed information about navigating health care insurance and costs. We do recommend using the resources of knowledgeable social workers, elder care coordinators, and lawyers.

We do not claim to know all the answers or have a crystal ball to predict the future. Any advice given in this book is based on our experiences with other people. It is practical and not clinical and not meant to replace care by your health care providers. Our own beliefs and values about life and death inform our thinking. They may not be the same as many who read this book. What we want to share is our voice of experience that we hope will assist you and your family as you navigate the difficult task of providing health care for yourself as you age and for your elderly loved one. While we tried to make each section focus on one issue, many of the ideas in each section are interlocking and build on material in other chapters. This reflects the complexity of the real life situations we all face.

Jane and Samuel Brody

2012

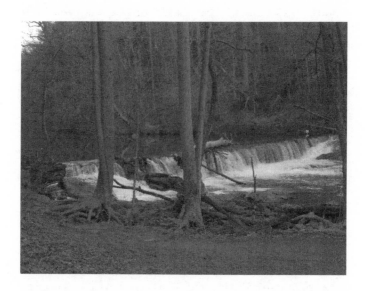

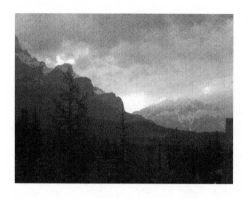

For everything there is a season,
a time for every purpose under heaven.
A time to be born and a time to die;
a time to plant and a time to pluck up that which is
planted;
a time to kill and a time to heal;
a time to break down, and a time to build up;
a time to weep and a time to laugh;
a time to mourn and a time to dance;
a time to cast away stones, and a time to gather
stones together;
a time to embrace and a time to refrain from
embracing;
a time to seek and a time to lose;
a time to keep, and a time to cast away;
a time to tear and a time to sew;
a time to keep silent and a time to speak;
a time to love and a time to hate;
a time for war and a time for peace.

Ecclesiastes 3:1-8 (World English Bible)

11

On A Personal Note from Sam:
The Case of the Social T's.

  Loss is universal. Experiencing loss is individual. The first loss I remember occurred when I was a sophomore in high school. Our school required that we each participate in what was loosely called community service. There were many options and, like much of what happens in life, I randomly chose to volunteer in a nursing home near our school because of its location. I could walk there. I was assigned to a man in his eighties who could no longer feed himself. In retrospect this was ironic since eating is one of my great joys.

  During one of my visits, I learned that he liked to snack on Social T crackers so I decided that next time I would bring him a box. When I arrived for my weekly visit, T's in hand, I was informed by the nurse that my patient had died. I may have helped this person only a handful of times, but I started looking forward to going and, on that day, I had brought him a special treat. He was so frail he could no longer feed himself. He was over eighty when death should not be unexpected. I had experienced the deaths of two of my grandparents and my father was a doctor so sickness was not a stranger. Still, I was surprised and saddened. Death caught me off-guard. For the loved ones of those at the end of life this is frequently their state of mind.

Section One: Assessing the Situation

"Should I Come?"

With their families so geographically dispersed, many elderly people live alone and far away from their closest relatives. An older adult could have multiple chronic physical problems which create a continuing cycle of declining and improving health status over a period of months and even years. Or the older adult could have one significant physical problem which leads to a sudden severe decline in health. The first cycle can be very wearing for family who keep traveling distances to visit their older sick family member as their health status waxes and wanes. The second scenario catches off guard those who only think of their elderly family member in their stable chronic state.

Sometimes families that are at a distance do not appreciate the level of deterioration in their family member because superficially things seemed to have remained the same or at least nothing has gone terribly wrong. Because family members may not have an accurate idea of how their loved one is doing on a daily basis and were not there for the recent change (whether rapid or gradual), it is hard for them to determine if this particular event requires them to come.

Sam had a patient, Larry Wilkins, who had a stroke in his late fifties which left him in constant pain. A device to infuse analgesic medication directly into his central nervous system was implanted. The problem was that the difference between providing comfort and overdose was very small. As he aged into his seventies, episodes of overdose began to occur. About twice a year he would end up in the emergency department (ED) in a coma. If a physician did not know Larry's history, he would think Larry had had another stroke and was at the end of life. Several times the overdose did almost kill him. He had to be admitted to the intensive care unit and put on a ventilator. But every time with supportive care, he came back to his baseline. Initially, his very supportive family came whenever he went to the ED. After several trips, they began to ask, "Should we come? Is it serious?" For Sam the problem became that even after multiple experiences with these overdose occurrences, he could never be certain any particular episode would resolve as positively for Larry as the previous ones had.

There are many thoughts and feelings implied in the question, "Should I come?" One is "Do I really need to come?" and expresses frustration. Perhaps this family member has made the journey multiple times in the past only to find the patient on the mend or resistant to their concerns and efforts to help. The elderly may not even want family members to know they are hospitalized because they do not want to be a burden or they do not want their family to interfere. Perhaps, this current health problem grew out of the patient's resistance to getting needed help or refusing reasonable care and the elder is trying to avoid "I told you so." The frustration, anger, and guilt of the family from past experiences may make them reluctant to enter into the health care decision process again. There can be infighting as one member blames the other for the elder's decline.

"Should I come?" may also be requesting a justification for not coming. In a sense the family is asking, "Can you handle this without me?" The family wants to be able to shift the responsibility for not being there to the physician. "The doctor didn't think it was so serious. He didn't say I should come." They do not want to be seen as uncaring or to feel guilty if the older person dies without their making an effort to visit, but they really do not want to make the trip.

The family may not be ignoring the patient but may have many other obligations and may need to prioritize the demands placed on them. Their own health may not be the best. Expenses in traveling long distances can be a burden. Getting the physician to let them pass on this one trip is a relief. If they believe that their loved one is getting good care and that their input into decision making is not that critical and can be done by telephone, they may choose to wait and see how things develop before coming.

"Should I come?" implies the question "Is it serious?" Sam has had experiences when the older adult has been brought to the emergency room and admitted to an intensive care unit and still family members will ask, "Is it serious?" Here "serious" usually means "life threatening." In the older adult, especially one who has a poor health baseline, determining which particular event will be the deciding event is not easy. We have had several patients who were close to death multiple times and who came back to live for months or longer (albeit with significant health problems). Other patients come in for a rather simple common illness, and in a domino fashion, one problem leads to another problem and finally death.

"Should I come?" may also mean "Is this the end?" Most people do not want their family member to die alone or among strangers. They want to offer the reassurance of a familiar face. They want to provide support and comfort. Some may also feel a need to say things that have until then been left unsaid or to say "I love you," one more time. Geographical distance does not mean emotional distance. Despite the miles between them, older adults and their family may feel quite connected and work hard to maintain their relationship. It is difficult not to come even when we think it is more likely that this will not be the final few days. Sam never tells family members not to come. He will clearly describe the current situation and the likely prognosis.

The key point to be taken away from this discussion is the great benefit that is derived from the elder having a long term relationship with a primary care provider and including a family member in that relationship—even if only by telephone. This keeps everyone up to date on the patient's current health status so when changes happen it is easier to make decisions. The primary care provider then knows the family from past encounters and communication is improved.

"She's Been Doing Fine until Now."

Loretta Scott was an 87 year old widow who lived in the same apartment for 58 years. She had a difficult year after her husband died, but rebounded and was able to create a satisfactory independent lifestyle for herself with friends, neighbors, and family. She had one daughter who lived about an hour away, called every day, and visited once or twice a month. Her other daughter lived in Europe and called every week.

During the past few years, her circle of friends and neighbors with whom she had contact had shrunken. She did not complain about this but continued to live simply in her apartment. Recently she started having a series of small difficulties. She tired more easily so stayed in the apartment alone. Arthritic pain interrupted her sleep and her appetite was diminished so she lost weight. She also was having some memory problems and was inconsistent in taking her medications for hypertension (high blood pressure) and heart disease. She never discussed these issues with anyone including many of the physicians she visited until she started seeing Sam who questioned her specifically about these very issues. (A geriatrician, the physician for the elderly, is trained to look at the functionality of the older adult just as a pediatrician tracks a youngster's growth and development.)

After completing a history and physical and with Loretta's approval, Sam called her local daughter to discuss some of his concerns about Loretta's declining status. Her daughter was initially surprised since she thought her mother was doing well. Sam told her to check her mother's medications and food; to closely observe her getting out of a chair or into the shower; to look at her financial records; and to take her out for a quick shopping trip to see how she tolerated it. Loretta's daughter called Sam back and expressed feeling guilty at how much she had assumed and not really assessed.

Many times Sam will speak to family members of an older adult who appears to them to have a sudden decline in health and functioning. They often seem bewildered by the abrupt change in status and say, "But she was looking so good." Sam uses the metaphor of water rising behind a dam to explain the process. If you are on the dry side of the dam, you really cannot know what is happening on the other side. Is the water going down or rising? Is it surging or quiet? Is it near the top? On the dry side of the dam, nothing changes until the conditions on the other side are critical and water spills over.

It can be hard to accurately assess the health and functional status of an older adult, especially if they are living alone. They may be aware of their decline but ashamed, fearful, or too stubborn to discuss it with others. They do not want others meddling, do not want to be a burden, and want to keep their independence. They may be unaware of how much they have declined because they have kept compensating for their deterioration in small steps. They may see the decline as normal for their age so not worth mentioning. They may become so accepting of their new limitations that they do not realize how vulnerable they have become. Cognitive impairment may impede judgment.

If family interaction is mostly by telephone or infrequent visits, the older adult may be able to "rise to the occasion" and perform temporarily at a higher level during the visit. It is easy to overlook subtle changes or explain a negative event as a freak occurrence. No one wants to admit that a loved one is failing.

Having a primary care physician who really knows the older adult is very important if the children are not near enough to carefully monitor their parent's condition. Because if a health emergency happens and the children are unaware of their parent's decline and the physician does not know the elder well, planning care is difficult. What is the patient's current baseline level of functioning? What safety issues need to be addressed before discharge? Do the patient and the family agree on the important issues? Having a physician who knows the patient and the patient's history well, can fill in much needed information when the family cannot.

Some elderly people have children who are still very emotionally and otherwise dependent on them. The limitations of adult children may interfere with their ability to develop a realistic perception of their parents. We have seen many elderly parents (mostly mothers) who in their eighties are still providing care to their children with psychiatric, cognitive, and addictive disorders. The issue is not providing support to enhance the elder's independence. The issue is getting the adult children help so they can function without depending on their elderly parents.

This is an extremely difficult area for intervention. A lifetime of caregiving is not easily changed. Even when it is obvious that the elderly parents cannot continue to provide care, the adult children will become angry and anxious about being "abandoned." They will resist and sabotage efforts to decrease their dependency on their parents. Intensive legal and social services, psychiatric care, family support, and "tough love" may be necessary to accomplish this goal.

"He Looked So Much Better Than Last Year"

Jane cared for a man in his early 90's who was in the late stages of dementia. Jack Sherman had been a lawyer and political leader in his community for over 50 years before cognitive decline forced him into retirement. At this point in his life, he could no longer communicate. He could not follow commands, was incontinent, and had to be fed. He could walk only with great assistance. His elderly brother took care of him at home with minimal help. One day Mr. Sherman fell on his brother, Thomas, who fractured his foot. Mr. Sherman was in a nursing home and his brother in a rehabilitation facility. It was unlikely that Thomas would ever be able to take care of Mr. Sherman at home again. When Mr. Sherman was hospitalized because of a fever, Jane met his niece who came every evening to feed him. She told Jane, "My uncle looks so much better now than he did last year." This statement surprised Jane. When she asked what this meant the niece talked about the list of acute health problems that plagued Mr. Sherman in the prior year.

Unlike the metaphor of water rising behind a dam in which problems are not yet observable until they literally spill over this is an example of a glacial perception on health (See "She's Been Doing Fine Until Now"). A glacier is massive, relentless, and progressive. Nothing really stops the

22

downward movement of a glacier (except global warming), but the movement is so slow that it is imperceptible to most people. The glacier becomes the norm—the way things are—and change is unrecognized. It is only at its end in a bay, when big chunks fall off into the water that change is evident.

As health declines in small increments over long periods of time, it becomes hard for those closest to the change to recognize it. When the health status is severely compromised for an extended period, the recognition of the severity of the condition is diminished. This loving niece had seen her vital vibrant uncle become almost infantile in his needs and abilities. In addition, Mr. Sherman's living arrangements had undergone a tremendous and irrevocable shift. Yet all his devoted niece could see was that there were currently fewer acute health problems.

When you are on the dry side of the dam, you do not see the problems on the other side that could lead to a catastrophe. When you are close to the glacier, the small incremental changes are almost unrecognized. The problem with both the water behind the dam and the glacier experiences is that people get lulled into thinking things are all right or at least stable. Proactive measures are not taken. Communication is limited and fails to address the real issues. Safety becomes compromised.

Proactive measures that should be done include the completing/updating of wills and advanced directives. Implementation of safety measures in the house is critical. These include structural alterations such as grab bars in the bathroom, walk-in tubs, installing better lighting, chair lifts, and moving bedrooms to the first floor. Other modifications that help with safety are the removal of throw rugs and acquiring emergency call devices. Education may help the older adult and the caregiver adapt better to the changes in functional status. Learning how to properly use a walker (those with built is seats are a plus) and hearing aids and other devices to amplify the sound on the telephone and television are not only safety measures but improve the quality of life.

Those who care for the elder need to meet with the health care providers, social services, legal resources, clergy, and others involved in caregiving to honestly discuss what is going on and what options are available. Developing a stronger support system will benefit both the elder and the caregivers.

"She should live another 20 years."

For several years Sam cared for a wonderful woman, Muriel Katz, who had been remarkably healthy in mind and body until well into her nineties. She came to America after WWII, married, and was able to see her daughter become a successful health care executive. Now she was experiencing the frailties and general decline that come with extreme old age. Despite what treatments modern medicine had to offer, there was nothing which would prevent the continued downward progression of her aging body. She had made peace with her situation but her only child, an unmarried daughter who had remained quite close to her mother and could be considered a senior citizen herself, refused to accept this.

One technique Sam uses when talking with families about treatment options and prognosis is to ask, "How long do you see your loved one living?" This is a gentle way to begin looking at end of life issues by laying a foundation for the realistic expectations needed in the discussion about how to make these last years the best possible. Most people when thinking about a ninety year old will say a few years. Some have the goal of their loved one reaching the major milestone of 100 years.

When making decisions about health care, thinking about age and life expectancy should enter the picture only as one of the variables. After the age of 70, how healthy an older person is will reflect more on the overall quality of life and level of function than age. The care provided a relatively healthy active 90 year old may not differ much from the care for a much younger person.

Conversely, the choices made for a person in their early 70's with severe neurological impairment and limited functioning should look quite different from the choices made for healthy seventy year olds because their needs are very different. In the former cases the best course of action is good supportive care, continued treatment of chronic health problems, and the avoidance of major complications such as falls and resulting hospitalizations.

A frail elderly person reaches the state when these supportive and preventative measures are not enough to maintain the patient's health, a decision must be made about how to proceed. For both the underlying chronic health problems and the acute conditions that arise, aggressive treatments that would be better tolerated in younger people are likely to result in more pain and suffering in the older adult.

The term aggressive is very emotional and value laden. But it must be acknowledged that many interventions such as surgery, chemotherapy, and mechanical ventilation, come with high risks for iatrogenic (health care caused) complications as well as increased pain and suffering. In our experience, intensive health care in the frail elderly is unlikely to achieve an extended period of good quality of life. Again the term good quality is value laden and may have different meaning for different people. Pain, immobility, nausea, lack of appetite, loss of independence, loss of privacy, and social isolation are all factors that influence a person's perception of "quality of life." (The issue of quality of life is discussed in more detail in the section, "Is It Worth It?")

For example, just keeping an intravenous line going for fluids and medications may require frequent multiple sticks in an elderly person with poor veins. If the person is confused, restraints which are frightening and demeaning may be applied to prevent the person from pulling out the intravenous line. The insertion of large intravenous access lines increases the risk of a life threatening infection because the elderly have weaker immune systems which make them more vulnerable to infections.

Often the choices between aggressive acute care and quality of life become contradictions in terms. The more you do to achieve one goal, the less you can do to achieve the other. Because of this contradiction, making decisions becomes much more complex. This is a major reason why advanced directives and discussion about them with your loved ones is so critical. (This issue is discussed in more detail in the section, "More is not Always Better.")

The thought of a loved one's death is frightening to most people, even as their loved ones reach the age of "life expectancy" and beyond. Although nothing will eliminate the feelings of fear and abandonment, having a discussion about values, beliefs, and goals regarding health care and end life issues can be extremely helpful.

In this story, Mrs. Katz's daughter who had been a health care provider herself prior to her administrative position, answered the question, "How long do you see your 94 year old mother living?" with the statement, "Twenty years." Did she actually think her mother would live to be 114? No, we do not think so. What she was saying was the thought of her mother dying was too frightening to accept. The daughter was in her late sixties. Perhaps the 20 years unconsciously represented how long the daughter thought she would live and she did not want to live without her mother. While these feelings and fears are very understandable and natural, they prevented her from accurately assessing her mother's health status and prognosis. This in turn prevented her from making decisions that would best serve her mother by preserving her mother's dignity and minimizing suffering.

Mrs. Katz had some mild cognitive decline but would still have been deemed competent. It appeared she went along with her daughter's wishes for more intensive treatment mostly to placate her daughter. She rallied, went home for a few months, but then her health deteriorated on multiple levels. Over the next 8 months there was a progression of acute episodes from which she would never completely recover. Although there were a few good days, they became fewer and farther apart. Finally, ten months after the initial conversation about how long her daughter thought her mother would live, Sam was able to get permission to refer Mrs. Katz to hospice. With his support and the support of the hospice staff, Mrs. Katz's daughter sadly accepted that her mother's life was nearing its end. Without the stress of repeated trips to the emergency department, hospitalizations and intensive treatment, Mrs. Katz died quietly in her apartment having just turned ninety-five.

"Looking at the Big Picture, Am I Too Old for This?"

Although many of our stories are about choosing health care options other than high tech acute care interventions, the following vignettes reflect the opposite course of action and when it is appropriate. When deciding how far to proceed with aggressive treatment, we continue to reinforce the need to look at the big picture--not just the person's age and current health problem and treatments. The patient's overall health status and quality of life, the patient's values and goals, and the patient's ability to recover from the effects of treatment and hospitalization must be considered.

Longer life expectancy has led to a significant increase in the population of elderly people in America. Some of this longevity has been related to advances in health care and environmental factors. Lifestyle changes with decreasing levels of smoking and better diet (except in the case of obesity and diabetes) have played a role. Good luck and great genes have helped those who have been able to live into their eighties without significant illness. However, even the most fortunate people cannot avoid the effects of aging forever. In the well elderly somewhere between ages 85 and 95, frailness impacts the quality of life even if there are no significant disease processes going on.

When patients in the 80's and 90's ask Sam, "Am I too old for this?" his response will be based on much more than their age. The patient may be asking about whether to undergo an extensive operation or may be inquiring about whether to take a trip overseas to see family on a special occasion. This is where looking at the big picture comes into play. Age alone should not be the determining factor. Functionality, stamina, and mental capacity must also be taken into account. Personal and social factors including support systems must be considered.

If the person is contemplating surgery or other invasive treatment, the risks, benefits, and alternatives should be carefully explored related to this patient's current status. Sam has had patients in their 80's who have done beautifully with open heart surgery and gained a better quality of life and a longer life. Knee and hip replacements can make substantial improvements by decreasing pain, increasing mobility, and enhancing socialization. A creative man with Parkinson's Disease who could no longer swallow efficiently, regained weight and energy after the placement of a permanent feeding tube.

If the person wants to travel, will the use of a wheelchair or other assistive devices be acceptable? Is there someone who can accompany the person who is capable of providing needed

31

help? How important is this trip to the person and family? Does the family have a plan if the elder's health declines while traveling? As with the decision about having surgery, the patient and family clearly need to delineate the pros and cons of travel while looking realistically about what will be demanded of the elder while traveling.

As a master's student working with the psychiatric liaison nurse at a university hospital, Jane met an elderly woman with peripheral vascular disease who had undergone repeated vascular surgeries for her problems. She was again experiencing circulatory blockage but was frustrated, worn out, and refused any more treatment. The surgeons called in the psychiatric team to evaluate the patient. Initially, Jane believed requesting a psychiatric consult showed disrespect for the patient's autonomy. However, when the psychiatric team evaluated the patient, they believed she was clinically depressed and suggested treatment with antidepressant medication. With treatment for the depression, the patient's mood improved, she became more optimistic, consented to treatment, and improved physically.

This highlights another point. We want to make decisions that respect the elder's autonomy, but we need to be careful to really talk and listen to the older adult and see what is truly motivating the decision — especially if it is a refusal of care.

Sometimes people will refuse treatment because their quality of life is so poor. Every effort should be made to improve appetite, sleeping, mobility, sensory functioning, and pain management before committing to a course of minimal treatment. Are they afraid of being a burden? Are they afraid of financial complications? Are they depressed? We want to be sure they can give informed consent— know the risks, benefits, and the alternatives. The woman with peripheral vascular disease could have refused to take the antidepressant. The fact that she agreed to psychiatric treatment was an additional indication that she wanted to get better.

We know of two women in their middle seventies who were healthy and active professionally and socially. Both received cancer diagnoses that in most cases would be considered terminal in a relatively short period of time. Both chose complicated surgical procedures in hopes of not just gaining time but curing the cancer. Both did very well initially and several years later are healthy and remain active professionally and socially.

When thinking about what course of action to take one thing to consider is the bigger picture which includes asking, "How frail is the older adult?" Some people like the two men above will probably be vibrant and strong well into their late 80's. Other people, especially those who had occupations that greatly taxed their bodies, may become frail in their 60's. For some people frailty will creep in slowly. For others it will seem to change a person in a matter of months. No matter what, frailty is part of the aging process.

An exact definition of frailty is hard to find. It includes a significant loss of independence in functioning and diminished overall health. Signs and symptoms of frailty include: weight loss, muscle mass loss, malnutrition, osteoporosis, impaired mobility, depression, decreased overall cognitive ability, and impaired immunity. It is related to level of function rather than specific diagnoses.

Balance and gait disturbances (related to osteoarthritis and neuromuscular decline) make the risk for falls and injury greater. Insomnia and other sleep disturbances further intensify symptoms. The old elderly experience losses of friends and family that can lead to depression and social isolation. Sensory losses (especially vision and hearing) become more pronounced which increases social isolation, impairs communication, and creates anxiety about leaving home. Many of the old old become housebound. Even those people who still desire to get out of their homes usually have decreased ability to do so. The inability to drive may accentuate these difficulties.

All of these functional losses and their accompanied emotional stress decrease the ability to perform the Instrumental Activities of Daily Living (IADL). These are activities such as shopping, cooking, laundry, housekeeping, and managing medication and finances which are necessary for people to live safely and independently within the community. Many of these actions reflect executive function which is the ability to plan, organize, and manage complex activities. (See Table on Levels of Dementia p. 189)

It is important to assess the elderly's ability to perform the IADLs. Check their finances. Are their bills being paid? Are they being scammed by some con artist who preys on the elderly? Check their cupboards and refrigerators. Is there enough food? Is it nutritious? Is it expired? Do the same in the medicine cabinet. Look at their clothing to see the condition of their shoes and apparel. Are they clean and serviceable? If you do not make a point of looking closely, it is possible to miss the beginning signs of decline. If your older adult refuses to let you make such an assessment, do the best you can without being intrusive and accept it. (See "You May Have to Accept that All You Can Do is to Pick up the Pieces.")

The good news is that with a variety of support services such as meal delivery and part time home health aides, the elderly can be maintained in their homes longer. There are different residential options such as assisted living that allow the older adult more privacy and independence while receiving needed support.

Declining function in the elderly will additionally impact on the Activities of Daily Living (ADL). These are more basic skills such as bathing and other hygiene tasks (oral care, shaving), dressing (clean and appropriate for the season), eating, toileting (continence) and transferring (a mobility issue related to being able to get out of bed or out of a chair). When a person reaches this stage, much greater intervention and support is needed to keep the person safe and foster as much independent function as possible.

Often frailty goes unrecognized until an acute illness or accident occurs. Then people expect that acute treatment will rectify all the health problems including those related to frailty. While acute care may help with the immediate illness or injury, acute care will have much less impact on frailty. Since frailty is a chronic often progressive condition, hospitals are not the best environments for interventions related to frailness. Imposed bedrest, lack of sleep due to noise, decreased nutrition, and a strange environment, magnify frailty.

Finally, although there may be no ongoing major chronic health problem when people reach the frail elder stage, any acute and relatively minor health problems can have serious implications. The frail elderly have less reserve and are less likely to "bounce back" after even relatively minor surgeries and injuries. Although much of this sounds depressing, accepting reality and dealing effectively with issues and problems will minimize some of the negative consequences. We say this to provide a backdrop against which health care decision making becomes more realistic and beneficial. Unclear understanding of your loved one's current health status or unreasonable expectations for your loved one's future may lead you to choices that do not achieve your goal--the best health care possible.

Jane remembers working with a physician who took pride that he "never gave up" on any of his patients. No matter how old, no matter how sick, no matter how poor the quality of their lives, he was always choosing the most aggressive course of action. One woman was in her 80's and had dementia from advanced Parkinson's Disease. She had resistant infections and was in an isolation room. She received feedings through a PEG tube (Percutaneous Endoscopic Gastrostomy tube through the skin into the stomach) and had a central venous line for all the antibiotics she was receiving. Her skin was beginning to break down and her kidneys to fail. Despite all these incurable problems, her physician would not consider palliative (comfort, symptom relief, and stress reduction care) or hospice care. The doctor kept treating each new complication totally out of context of the big picture. The family was unquestioning and agreed to whatever the physician said.

Assessment by a geriatrician is important because geriatricians (physicians who specialize in the care of the elderly) are trained to look at the special needs of the elderly in a broader scope than many general internists. Based on this assessment, holistic and realistic care can be planned and provided. Flexibility in the use of varied resources such as physical medicine, rehabilitation and subacute settings, long term care, and home care is important. Most geriatricians use palliative care principles to enhance the quality of life by focusing on comfort measures such as pain and symptom management in addition to curative measures. They understand the conflicting desires to keep the elder at home and provide for safe care.

Studies have shown that older adults who receive strong supportive home care services have fewer emergency department visits and re-hospitalizations. High rates of re-hospitalization and emergency department visits reflect poor management of care at the end of life. Most older adults prefer to remain at home.

"Things Change"

In general and when working with the elderly, it is important to remember that things can change radically in a short period of time. There can be tremendous shifts in the person's physical and mental status. Unanticipated or hoped-to-be-avoided injuries and complications occur. The social support system that keeps older adults functioning at their highest level may be overwhelmed or damaged. We emphasize this point because the advice you receive from your health care provider one day may not fit the situation on another. Your goals and plans should be frequently reassessed and may need to be adjusted.

Jessica Bryons was a woman in her mid-80's who had a history of multiple abdominal surgeries beginning with caesarian sections for the delivery of her three children. The last abdominal surgery for a bowel obstruction (inability of food to pass through the gastrointestinal tract) was fraught with complications and she nearly died. Now she was fully recovered and residing comfortably in an assisted living facility. However she was very troubled by the large hernia that developed at the site of her last abdominal surgery. The sight of it made her depressed and anxious. She did not like this disturbance in her body image and decided to have surgery to repair the hernia.

Sam saw her for pre-operative clearance. Although she had some chronic health issues, she was in good shape for her age. The hernia was causing no physical complaints. (The biggest threat with a hernia is that a loop of bowel could get trapped and twisted in the opening in the abdominal wall. This can lead to bowel obstruction, or even worse, cut the blood supply to that loop of bowel causing death to the tissue.) As part of the visit Sam reviewed her past poor experiences with surgery and discussed the possibility that abdominal surgery yet again could lead to more problems with healing and support of the abdominal organs. After talking to her and her son who accompanied her, she decided to reconsider whether to go through with the operation. As a general rule, the older a person gets, the more elective surgical procedures should be avoided. This is especially true for people with chronic health problems such as diabetes, COPD (chronic obstructive pulmonary disease such as emphysema), and heart disease.

Ironically and unfortunately, two days after seeing Sam, Jessica Bryon's hernia became caught and twisted. The surgery was no longer elective. She did well with the operation and recovered without incident. Was Sam too cautious? He had seen too many people do poorly with unnecessary surgery and gave his best advice. Yet in the end, each person is different and no one can exactly predict what will happen.

Bill and Ruth Just provide another example of how things change. Bill and Ruth had done well financially. They sold the business they started from scratch for a tidy sum when Bill turned sixty five, seventeen years ago. They lived in their 4,000 square foot detached 3 story home for the past forty one years. None of their four children and nine grandchildren lived nearby so until two years ago they spent at least two months a year traveling to visit--usually staying a week but sometimes more-- with one child or another.

Four years ago Bill broke his hip in a skiing accident and although he seemed to make a full recovery, decided to put down the skis permanently. Still he and Ruth remained active both physically and mentally. They were regularly seen walking through their neighborhood and both took senior oriented exercise classes twice a week at the local Y. About two years ago Ruth thought she might be having some memory problems. She had not told Bill, but on several occasions had driven to the grocery store only to forget what she wanted to buy. About a week before her medical visit she became frightened when she got lost driving home from the Y. A concerned police officer led her back home, but made her promise to at least tell her doctor about what happened.

"Is it Alzheimer's, Doctor Brody?" Memory testing, scans, and blood tests showed that she was in the early stages of dementia (There is no specific test for AD. See "Always a Step Behind"). Since Alzheimer's is the most common cause of dementia in the United States, she was probably correct. Sam asked her to schedule a follow up visit with her husband so they could discuss the results.

Sam had known Bill and Ruth for over fifteen years. They trusted him. "Looks like Ruth's in the early stages of dementia. There is no sign of any other cause, Ruth, so we need to start your care for this condition."

"You mean medication. I've read there are medicines for this but it doesn't look like any of them help that much. What do you think?"

"There's more than just the medicine."

Over the next few months Sam met with Ruth, Bill, and several of their children. Thankfully, this wonderful couple was willing to discuss all the issues including the fact that it was hard to predict how rapidly Ruth would decline. At one of the meetings Ruth told Bill that she never wanted to leave the house.

"Don't put me away. Let me die at home."
Sam heard it and hoped she could have her wish but
things got complicated when Bill fell down the
basement stairs and re-fractured his hip. He was
taking care of most of the household chores at that
point with only a once a week housekeeper to do the
heavy cleaning. He would need surgery and then
weeks of rehabilitation. His fall and the fracture
also meant that for this once vibrant man, now in
his eighties, the future was very uncertain. It was
unlikely he would be able to continue to be the
primary care-giver for his wife whose dementia was
now in the moderate stage.

She no longer drove and needed help
preparing meals, dressing, and with some toileting
activities. Their son, Rodney, lived closest and
came immediately. It would take several days to
organize Ruth's care. Rodney arranged for their
housekeeper to stay during the day while he visited
local assisted living facilities and began calling
some of the numbers Sam gave him regarding other
home-care options. Money was not the issue for the
Justs but ensuring Ruth's safety, medical care, and
need for socialization were all part of Rodney's
journey. After meeting with several geriatric care
managers, he decided to keep Ruth home with 24
hour help. He would start with two, twelve hour
shifts as her sleep cycle often found her up in the
middle of the night. He also signed her up to attend
the adult day care program at their church.

Sam told Rodney that this initial plan was excellent. He could already see that Bill's absence was very disturbing for Ruth. She had more frequent episodes of agitation which in the past Bill could usually manage with a comforting hand and a stroll outside. Sam met with Ruth's caregivers to discuss techniques for avoiding agitation and how to handle agitation when it occurred. Everyone decided to leave medication as a last resort but realized it might be needed.

Bill returned home after six weeks in rehabilitation. His spirit was strong but he had become quite frail. He walked with a walker and needed to rest frequently. The Justs needed all the help Rodney and the other children had arranged. However after six months at home, Bill decided he would take a look at several of the assisted living facilities near Rodney's home. There was a beautiful facility on a lake. The director was an avid skiing buff so he and Bill immediately connected. The Justs moved to Overbridge a month later. Ruth was placed on a special unit for persons with more advanced dementia and Bill had his own room near the computer library. When Ruth's condition declined a year later, she was moved to the facility's hospice where she died with Bill by her side.

This encapsulated story condenses many years of caregiving and highlights some key points:

- Be prepared to modify plans. Better yet, plan ahead for changes. Making decisions in a rush will be less likely to provide the best results.

- Think about avoiding or limiting stairs, transportation accessibility, and other factors important to you if you are downsizing. One living situation may work at one point but not forever.

- Try it out. Be open to new ways of doing things. If you don't like it or it does not work, try something else. Do not say, "This is the way I've always done it."

- Speak with financial advisors and elder care lawyers to find out how to maximize your assets. It is important to find out what you can afford.

Section Two: Safety

"Always One Step Behind"

A friend of ours whose mother developed dementia from Alzheimer's Disease (AD) not long after Sam's father died from the same illness said, "The best thing you ever said to me was that the family was always one step behind in adjusting to the decline in functioning of their loved one with dementia." This is something we found true in both our personal and professional experience. Often without even realizing it, families adapt to the slow decline seen in dementia by assuming more and more of the tasks the person with AD can no longer perform around the house or in social situations. They rationalize that what is happening is only normal aging. Cognitive deficits are written off as jokes about "senior moments" or result of stress, fatigue, or stubbornness.

Sam's mother slowly increased the amount of talking she did for his father who as a psychiatrist had been very verbal and people-centered. Initially it was not obvious what she was doing to anyone, even her. It happened gradually and without planning. Also, although Sam's father may not have recognized with whom he was speaking, a lifetime of strong communication skills saw him through many social situations. He had stock phrases--"How's your family?" "Well, that's how it goes," and "It's been a pleasure talking to you"-- that made it seem like he actually understood what was said and knew with whom he was talking. Even in the very late stages of dementia, people could talk to him for several minutes at some social function and then come to us and accuse us of making things sound worse than they were. In fact two weeks before he died at home in hospice, the hospice nurse was discussing the possibility of him removed from home hospice care. Between Sam's mother's heroic efforts to keep him looking as good as possible and his father's charm, it was easy to overlook the deficits.

The erosion in functioning may be so subtle and gradual that it goes unrecognized. No one wants to think the unthinkable. Some patterns are labeled as personal quirks or foibles. For example, "Dad always forgot that he put the teakettle on the stove." Sam's father had burnt through three kettles before Sam's mother took the knobs off the stove to prevent him from turning it on. (Boiling water had always been the extent of his interest in cooking.) We had seen many patients who are well into the middle stage of AD whose families were shocked to learn the patient had dementia.

Often it is a change in the environment, like a hospitalization, that places the decline in focus for the first time. This is because patients with dementia are prone to become more confused and delirious when hospitalized than are older persons who do not have dementia. (See table below comparing delirium and dementia) People with AD are overwhelmed by new stimuli they cannot process. Anxiety increases and further diminishes cognitive and perceptual abilities. A response called a "catastrophic reaction" can occur and the patient becomes agitated and verbally and physically aggressive. This is one reason we all should strive to avoid hospitalization in the elderly especially those who have any form of dementia.

Comparison of Symptoms	
Delirium	**Dementia**
Rapid acute onset	Gradual insidious development
Quickly progressive—can lead to death	Slowly progressive—death usually from complication such as infection
Intense anxiety and irritability	Blunted or labile moods Anxiety and apathy
Insomnia, hyperactivity, and tremors	Decreased coordination and inability to perform basic skills (such as dressing)
Fever, fast heart rate, and high blood pressure	Memory loss—first short term then long term
Hallucinations	Impaired new learning and judgment
Convulsions	Loss of language skills

Denial is often the first defense against the recognition of decline. Sam's mother once asked the two of us and Sam's brother who is a psychiatrist if we thought Sam's father had Alzheimer's Disease. By this point he was in the middle stages of dementia. He had significant expressive aphasia (loss in ability to speak) as well as deterioration in many other areas of functioning. We all replied, "Unfortunately, yes." It was not the answer she wanted and she quickly discounted what we said. "Oh no, I think he just has some memory problems." More ways of rationalizing his decline occurred. To say Sam's father had a terrible sense of direction would be an understatement and he never was very invested in driving so Sam's mother throughout their marriage often did the driving. When the dementia progressed and she took over all of the driving it did not seem like a major event. Even when she could no longer deny that something was seriously wrong she would not utter what she called "The A-word."

Some friends cared for their mother, Lois Murphy, who had AD in their home. On weekends, other siblings and family members would occasionally stop by and visit. Lois who was always a quiet woman enjoyed sitting and watching everyone. When her care and safety needs exceeded what our friends could provide, they broached the subject of placement in a nursing home with their siblings. Their family was horrified and angry that they would do such a thing. Lois could not be that big of a problem. When our friends went away on a small vacation they had Lois stay with some of the other siblings. When they got back, the family began an open discussion about residential placement.

Alzheimer's Disease (AD) is the most common cause of dementia. It was once called presenile dementia when senility or dementia was viewed as normal aging and only a disease if it occurred early—prior to the age 65. Dementia is not normal aging. It just occurs at increasing rates as the elderly age.

It was discovered that the same physiological processes (deposits of plaques made of a protein—peptide β amyloid—and tangles in the neural fibers that transmit messages) were occurring in AD at whatever age the onset. These are presumed to be the causes of AD but this is still being debated. In addition, there is a reduction of the neurotransmitter acetylcholine. Although many people use the terms dementia and AD interchangeably, there are more than 50 possible causes of dementia besides AD. Vascular dementia (also called multi-infarct dementia) occurs when very small blood vessels in the brain become blocked leading to brain tissue death. This is the second most common cause of dementia. Unlike the slow steady decline seen in AD, vascular dementia often has a more step-like progression with periods of relative stability broken by short periods of rapid decline. It is not uncommon to have both AD and vascular dementia together.

Chronic thiamine (vitamin B-1) deficiency, often seen with alcoholism, can lead to a form of dementia known as Wernicke-Korsokoff Syndrome. Repeated head trauma that may occur in sports such as boxing or football can lead to dementia. Neurological diseases such as Parkinson's Disease and Multiple Sclerosis frequently cause dementia. There are genetic disorders such as Huntington's Disease (formerly known as Huntington's Chorea because of the muscle twitching that occurs as part of the disease process) that cause dementia. Dementia can be seen as part of an infection with HIV, the virus that causes AIDS.

All these dementias have their own specific clusters of symptoms and patterns of decline but all are progressive in their loss of cognitive function (*impaired judgment, memory loss, poor reasoning, disorientation, decreased attention, delusions, and apraxia—the inability to perform tasks such as working the microwave or tying shoes*), perception (*hallucinations*), language (*aphasia--ability to speak and understand language*), motor capabilities (*agitation, involuntary movements, poor coordination, decreased reflexes, muscle weakness*) and emotional health (*apathy, irritability, paranoia, depression, erratic feelings*). Overall, dementia is a regression of mental and physical abilities that occurs over many years.

The person with dementia will initially find methods to mask deficits. Sam's father kept a small notebook with information in it and had secretly purchased several books and tapes for memory enhancement which we discovered when clearing out his office. We wish he had felt able to talk to us about his fear and concerns, but by the time his dementia was apparent to his health care professional children, the discussion could not occur. One reason for this was that in his mid-70's Sam's father had surgery for an abdominal aortic aneurysm. His immediate post-operative course was very rocky and he developed delirium and was restrained. (Delirium is much more common in patients with dementia.) His anger and shame over this incident was profound. It took him almost a year to recover physically and emotionally and just as it seemed he was becoming his "old self", the symptoms of his advancing AD became apparent.

We sometimes reflect about whether it would have been better to forego the aneurysm surgery. The aneurysm was not that big and rupture was not that likely. If given the choice of the surgery, its aftermath, and the years or decline from AD or no surgery and a few good years until a sudden death, we think he would have chosen the latter. But as we said in the foreword, we have no crystal ball and he chose to have the surgery.

One problem in determining what situations are safe for a patient with dementia is that while the overall trajectory is one of decline, from day to day and even during the same day, there may be periods of better or much worse functioning. Sundowner's syndrome is a name given to the decreased cognitive functioning and increased agitation that occurs in the evening. When Jane was working the evening shift on a neurosurgical unit, older patients who were oriented and cooperative during the day would become confused and combative in the evening. Someone may look very good at a certain time or in a certain situation but be very disoriented and agitated at another time or in a different situation. Many people with dementia may seem fine when left alone 90% of the time. The problem is that no one can predict the 10% of time when problems will occur. In actuality, at this point they are not really that fine any of the time. They and their caregivers have been lucky that their deficits did not cause problems.

As Sam's father's health declined, we kept saying to each other, "Well, this is the bottom. He can't get any worse." Unfortunately he could and did. Thinking like this is one reason the caregivers are always a step behind the reality of the situation.

To clarify some points about caring for the person with dementia we want to discuss childrearing. When parenting classes are given to people with newborns, the parents are taught to be prepared for their child's developmental milestones and adjust what they are doing to keep their children safe. "Don't leave the newborn near the end of the bed because one day she will learn to roll over and could fall." "Take down the mobile from over your son's crib because he will soon be pulling up and could get tangled in it." "Move the cleaning products from beneath the sink or your child who has just learned to crawl will get into them." As parents we acknowledge our responsibility to keep our children safe. We look forward to each developmental milestone—walking, talking, toileting—as a positive sign of our child's health and growing capabilities.

The changes that occur throughout childhood are gradual but continuous. It is when someone has not seen a child for a period of time that the developmental growth seems pronounced. Those who see the child daily are less aware of the changes except for major advances such as pulling up and walking. The first words are noteworthy milestones while the later shift to speaking in sentences is less obvious. The parents are proud of their child's progress and are eager to tell others of each new accomplishment. Our young children may whine and complain (especially those terrible twos) but they do see us as authority figures and have no experience of being independent and autonomous. Also they are smaller than their parents.

Dementia is this whole process turned on its head. When someone has dementia, developmental functioning goes in reverse. Each loss is another reminder of declining health and capabilities and an omen of worse things to come.

We often ask families to relate the capabilities of their loved ones to that of a child of a certain age. For example, can they function as well as a 6 year old in getting dressed without assistance, following directions, problem solving, and maintaining their hygiene? If they are equal to a 6 year old, then the type of activities planned should reflect where they are developmentally for safety and to reduce anxiety. If family members would feel uncomfortable leaving a child with a similar developmental age without supervision (below babysitting age--developmentally of 13 or 14), they probably should not leave their elder alone. If they would not take a child of 6 to a fancy restaurant with slow service, it is probably not a good idea to do the same with an elder with the same developmental level. It is important to remember that the person's ability to process the environment is diminished. The fear of being inappropriate may cause anxiety in the elder and the family. Simple activities and routines will bring much more pleasure to the person with AD and those who provide care. When Sam's Dad could no longer follow the plots of most movies, he still enjoyed watching musicals.

As mentioned earlier, children know nothing except a world in which the adults provide the structure and rules. The older adult is accustomed to being independent and self-directed. The older adult with dementia may not perceive deficits and get angry when restrictions for safety are put into place. Giving up activities such as driving can cause significant changes in the elder's lifestyle which understandably he or she want to avoid. It also is a clear indication that decline has occurred. (The issue of declining abilities is discussed in more detail in the section, "I've Been Driving for Fifty Years Without an Accident.")

Another major safety issue is the agitation and acting out that can occur in elderly people with dementia, especially when they are frightened or anxious. Certainly a variety of environmental changes (routines, simplified familiar surroundings) and communication techniques (short sentences with nonverbal cues) can help decrease the periods of increased anxiety and acting out. These actions make working with the patient with dementia less stressful.

Caretakers and patients alike are at great risk for injury. It may seem easier for residential facilities and even with home care to medicate the patients as the first line of treatment. Patients may be medicated (and restrained) for staff needs rather than taking the time for non-pharmacological approaches. However, most of the medications have some risks and overmedication is common.

If these measures do not work then medication may be needed. Many older adults do not do well with the antianxiety and hypnotic (sleeping) agents such as the benzodiazipines: alprazolam (Xanax), diazepam (Valium), lorazepam (Ativan), and temazepam (Restoril) or antihistamines such as diphenhydramine (Benadryl). These drugs can easily cause oversedation and remain active for longer periods in the elderly. Overmedicating the elder creates a hosts of additional other problems such as poor nutrition because a person is too drowsy to eat. They also can cause hypotension and dizziness which increases the risks for falls. Some older adults experience a paradoxical excitement with the antianxiety agents that can lead to agitated and aggressive behavior. For chronic anxiety conditions, antidepressants such as [citalopram (Celexa) and venlafaxine (Effexor)] often work best. Medication decisions need to be discussed fully with the elder's health care provider.

The drugs of choice for agitation and severe anxiety usually are antipsychotics. These medications should be given in very small doses as the elderly are extremely sensitive to their effects. The goal should be to decrease the agitation but not to oversedate. There is a debate about the use of antipsychotics, also called neuroleptics and historically called major tranquillizers, to treat the agitation seen in dementia. This group of medications is approved to treat the psychosis seen in schizophrenia and also the agitation/psychosis seen in the manic stage of bipolar illness. Treating the agitation of dementia with antipsychotics is an off lable use—a use for a condition other than the one approved by Food and Drug Administration (FDA).

Recent research has indicated that the antipsychotics such as risperidone (Risperdal), quetiapine (Seroquel), or haloperidol (Haldol) which are used in the elderly to treat dementia agitation cause a slight increased mortality rates. In most cases we believe that if non-pharmacological measures have not reduced severe agitation, then keeping the patient and caretakers safe in the here and now takes priority. The doses should be started at very low levels and if need be increased in very small increment—"Start low, go slow." However, this is a decision every family must make for themselves after careful consideration.

"I've Been Driving for Fifty Years Without an Accident"

As discussed in "Always One Step Behind," trying to assess what is safe for a person with declining cognitive and motor function is difficult. One reason is that although the general direction of functioning is downward, there are temporary periods where the decline is not as evident and periods when functioning is significantly impaired. Also the decline tends to be progressive so constant reassessment is needed. What works now probably will not work later.

Many times when Sam introduces the subject of limiting some activity, the patients' first response is that they have been doing that activity for decades. "I've been driving for fifty years without an accident." "I've been climbing the stairs to my apartment for forty years." "I've been shoveling snow since before you were born." Sometimes Sam takes a humorous approach and talks about how he could jump and touch the basketball hoop when he was in high school—a very short lived phenomenon.

The resistance to the restrictions in activity is normal. We do not want to face that we cannot do what we once were able to do. Not being able to touch a basketball hoop is not much of a loss, but giving up driving is a significant change. Providing reasons for the change may help. But reasoning with a person with dementia is not effective. Reinforcing the strengths and capabilities that remain is helpful as is assisting the elder find ways to live with the new limitation in activity--senior rides, elevators, hiring local teens to shovel.

Driving differs from others areas of restriction because it not only affects the elder's safety but the safety of others. Driving in our culture is related to freedom and self-reliance. Many elders would be isolated without the ability to drive. Almost all teens look forward to getting their driver's license. Driving is probably one of the most contentious areas where restrictions may be needed. Losing permission to drive emphasizes the losses that occur with aging.

Visual and hearing impairments coupled with decreased reflexes can lead to unsafe driving. As people get more uncomfortable driving, their anxiety increases. Increased anxiety impairs perception and the ability to process information. This leads to more risk. Although people may remember the mechanics of how to drive, their ability to navigate and find where they want to go may decline.

Self-reports of driving ability are usually not reliable. When pressed many seniors will say, "Well, they renewed my license, so that must mean I can drive." Or "I only drive locally." During the later stages of dementia, the ability to see the loss in function is gone. Family and caregivers are usually more accurate in assessing whether a person is still safe to drive. However, Sam has patients with moderate dementia that drove to their initial workup.

The Family Caregiver Alliance (FCA) www.caregiver.org suggests a caregiver have the elder whose driving ability is in question to ride as the passenger and give instructions on what should be done regarding signaling, lane changes, speed, and traffic signs. This will highlight what the person is able to do or not do. The FCA also suggests having people with early stage or mild dementia evaluated by an independent driving instructor.

Because the process of dementia is progressive, even if someone passes the driving test initially, retesting should be performed every 6 months or when significant changes in functioning occur. People with moderate or severe dementia do not need to be tested as they should not be driving.

A person displays poor judgment, has fallen asleep at the wheel, has difficulty processing information, is easily agitated, or is less aware of surroundings, should not be driving. Driving behaviors that would be red flags include: driving slowly and hesitantly, avoiding left turns, and not signaling. No longer being able to drive in the rain or at night or having difficulty staying in traffic lanes, demonstrate significant driving impairment. If the elder has gotten lost while driving or has had a series of small "fender benders," driving has become too dangerous an activity.

Trying to reason with people whose dementia has progressed to the point they should not be driving is usually futile and frustrating. As we said earlier, people with dementia cannot appreciate the changes in functioning that have occurred. Telling them they may hurt someone else makes no sense to them since they think they are driving well and may not remember the conversation anyway.

Having the news come from a physician, independent driving instructor, or the Motor Vehicle Bureau may make the transition easier, but not always. In most states, physicians are not required to inform the Motor Vehicle Bureau of patients who they believe should not be driving.

Some times the urge to drive will be triggered by seeing car keys or the car itself. Once it has been determined that a person should no longer be driving, removing these visual reminders (parking the car around the corner or in a garage) may help with the transition. In many cases, people who adamantly refused to stop driving became adjusted to this new norm within a short period .

If a person can no longer walk 30 feet in a reasonable amount of time, his/her physical ability to drive is probably diminished. (Of course paraplegics can drive but their neurologic impaired is in the spine, not the brain). It is important to tell people, especially the health care providers, about the fact that this older adult is no longer driving. As Jane's father's post-polio syndrome worsened, he had to stop driving. He could not switch from the gas to the brake quickly enough. After not driving for a year, Jane's father asked his cardiologist if it was okay for him to drive. The cardiologist replied that her could, not considering his post-polio syndrome or that he had not driven for over a year. Fortunately, Jane's father never really reconsidered his decision.

Another issue that comes up is if one person stops driving who is going to take up the slack? Sometimes the spouse of the person who stops driving is barely able to drive. If the older adult lives alone, will children and other family members be available to drive to the store, the doctor, religious services, and friends? In urban areas, there is more within walking distance and taxis and other transportation are readily available. In suburban and rural areas, the loss of driving can create quite a hardship. As people get into their 80's, thinking ahead about how they will manage without driving is important. Moving into an area with more support usually make sense. This is a proactive decision the well elderly can do that will ease their transition as they age.

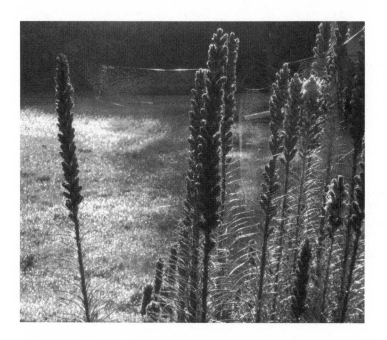

"You May Have to Accept that All You Can Do is To Pick up the Pieces"

Nothing can be more frustrating than trying to take reasonable steps to promote safety only to have the elder at risk resist. There are stereotypes of the elderly as "cute little old ladies," or "cantankerous old men with a heart of gold," but getting older does not often bestow a sudden improvement in personality. People who were difficult, demanding, and mean earlier in life carry those traits with them into older adulthood. As people age their underlying personality traits such as stubbornness or suspiciousness can become more pronounced. Ingrained cultural beliefs about not being a burden or "charity case," may cause an older adult to refuse needed help. Agitation and paranoia frequently accompany declining mental function. With an increased anxiety level, the ability to rationally discuss an issue becomes very limited. All of the above factors not only lead to unsafe living situations for the elder, they also make it more difficult to intervene.

Underlying family friction, sibling rivalry, and a history of accumulated slights—real and imagined, all come into play when families have to make decisions about their older adults. We have known families that have gone through great strife over something as simple as installing grab bars in the bathroom since the bars were an acknowledgement of physical decline that was being denied.

Jane cared for an elderly man who fell and lay on the floor for two days. His wife could not get him up but fed him and took care of him as he lay on the floor. It was not until one of their children popped in for a quick unannounced visit that he got the help he needed. This patient experienced severe complications from lying on the hard floor for two days. The breakdown of his muscle released substances damaging to his kidneys into the bloodstream. He developed decubiti (bedsores) that took a long time to heal. All of this could have been prevented if his devoted wife had called for help when he first fell.

Self-neglect is a term used to describe situations when the elderly do not seem to be adequately keeping themselves safe and healthy. This may include not following the prescribed health regimen, not using air conditioning on extremely hot days, poor hygiene, and inadequate nutrition. Self-neglect puts them at risk for serious injuries and additional health problems which could be prevented. Self-neglect tends to be progressive. When assessing for self-neglect, the caregivers and health care providers should look for underlying causes such as dementia, substance abuse, medication side effects/overdose, and depression. Because the deterioration into self-neglect is usually gradual, the elder may have become accustomed to a living situation which to an outsider would be intolerable.

It is very frustrating to deal with a loved one experiencing self-neglect. It seems so obvious to others what is wrong and what needs to be done to correct the problem. (When family members actually disagree about how severe the problem is and what should be done, this adds an additional layer of issues to navigate.) Many times the solutions seem relatively easy and non-intrusive. However, the older adults' perspective can be quite the opposite. Maintaining their independence, pride and not letting others know how poorly they are doing may be the priority.

They may see uninvited attempts to help as invasive and domineering. They may attribute bad motives (such as trying to steal from them) to unwanted efforts to change their situation. Some older adults refuse help because they fear the costs or do not understand the nature of the services offered. They may not want strangers--including visiting nurses, home health aides, and social service personnel—in their home. They may come across as unreasonable and inflexible.

The key point here is how unreasonable are they? We all have the freedom to make bad choices for ourselves. The law rightly insures that the elderly have the same right. As long as people are competent/ have capacity, they can make most decisions about how they live and the type of care they receive. Even if the elder's decision could lead to serious health consequences, if the elder has capacity/competence, his or her decisions must be accepted. So even if your mother has fallen a few times and is unsteady on her feet, you cannot force her to use a walker, wear an alarm, or go into assisted living. Unless their home violates a housing or sanitation code, the elderly have the right to stay in their home—even if it is dirty and in disrepair. As Sam will tell frustrated family members, "You may have to accept that all you can do is to pick up the pieces."

The only time anyone can override that freedom is when the elder is found to be incapacitated or incompetent. Having a loved one legally declared incapacitated or incompetent is wrenching, but may be needed to override the elder's unsafe choices. A geriatric neuropsychiatric examination should be performed. Getting the elder to participate in this examination may not be easy. Even if a finding of incapacity or incompetence is made, some self-neglecting elders may still refuse to cooperate or sabotage efforts to help.

Incompetency in the frail elderly is typically a permanent legal status. People are deemed to be incompetent if they are unable to manage their personal/financial affairs because of mental or physical disability. After evaluation by experts and a hearing, a judge will appoint a guardian or conservator to take charge of the personal/financial affairs. The guardian does not have to be the same as the person designated as the health care agent.

Incapacity is a more fluid, less permanent state in which a person is declared unable to make health care decisions for him or herself at that time. It is medically determined by two physicians who must examine the person and agree on the patient's decision making capacity. To be declared incapacitated a person must lack the ability to make informed decisions about his or her health— unable on at least a rudimentary level to weigh the risks, benefits, and alternatives. It does not mean the person is oriented to time and place or knows who the president is. It does not mean the person is free of psychiatric conditions. The depth of knowledge about the risks, benefits, and alternatives does not have to be extensive. A basic understanding of the situation (including the risks) and the ability to state a clear treatment choice is all that is required. If a person is found to lack capacity, then the agent identified in the advanced directive becomes the health care decision maker. If there is no advanced directive, the legally defined next of kin takes on that responsibility. (See section, "If I Don't Discuss it, I Won't Die," for more on this issue)

When people think about the elderly, issues of substance abuse are often neglected. Yet addicts and alcoholics do grow old. So some elderly people have long histories of substance abuse and may have significant health problems related to it—such as dementia from alcoholism. Also many older adults fall into alcohol and drug abuse after experiencing the loss and isolation of retirement and death of family and friends.

Sam had an elderly patient who occasionally had seizures. These were usually preceded by episodes when the patient had difficulty walking. After taking a careful history, Sam discovered that the patient was an extremely heavy drinker. When he was unable to go out and buy liquor, he experienced seizures, a severe alcohol withdrawal symptom.

Here are some suggestions for dealing with an elder who resists help:

- Call or visit frequently.

- Whenever possible try to validate the elder's concerns and values.

- Give recognition for some area where the elder is doing well.

- Try to offer choices when possible rather than come across as dictating.

- Give information about available support services, how they operate, and what benefits they provide. This may increase their acceptance.

- Ask them to try a service for a short time and promise to revisit the choice in a month.

- Make small acceptable changes as a place to start.

- Check their finances to be sure their bills are getting paid and they are not being scammed by some con artist

One point Sam frequently makes to a patient who is declining help is, "By taking this amount of help (hands showing a small space), you can retain this amount of independence (hands showing a wide space.) If you don't take any help, you are likely to get into a situation where your health will fail or you might get injured and you will require much more assistance." This is an idea family members should reinforce.

Some patients tell Sam, "If I fall and die, it's OK with me." Sam replies, "You may fall and not die but lie there in pain until someone discovers you." Surprisingly, almost everyone to whom Sam has said this did not consider the second possibility. Sam presents this information factually and nonjudgmentally which allows the elder to hear it with less defensiveness.

Threats and ultimatums will not work but this does not mean you cannot discuss the risks of certain behaviors. About one half of older adults who fall and have a broken hip will die within the year, Information such as this can lay a foundation for using a cane or walker, wearing sensible shoes, removing throw rugs and clutter, and installing grab bars and better lighting. As frustrating as the situation may be, it is important to keep the lines of communication open.

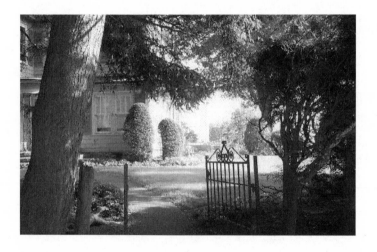

"More is Not Always Better"

As we age the two basic methods our bodies use to process and remove toxins—metabolism by the liver and excretion by the kidney—work less well. Liver and kidney function decline. Medications are eliminated by the body in the same manner as toxins and even at normal doses, drug levels can become toxic. The best rule for medicating the elderly is to "Start low and go slow." The older adult especially the very elderly (over age 85), need dosages to be less than in the younger adult. Also any increase in the dose should occur very gradually and in small increments.

This is a general rule and a practitioner skilled in working with the elderly will know when it is necessary break such a rule. For example, if a person has been on low doses of cortisone for a chronic problem such as arthritis, a brief period of much higher doses of cortisone may be needed to get the person through a stressful acute episode of an illness.

Knowing what to treat and how far to go is not easy to decide either. In the older adult the benefits of certain treatments, including medications, may be more limited while the risks increase for complications from the treatments. Even basic guidelines on when to treat need to be reconsidered and adjusted for the older individual.

For example, the current suggestion for treatment of hypertension is to keep the blood pressure below 140/90. Yet Sam has patients who get extremely weak, dizzy and faint if he medicates them to reach that point. They are active and happy with blood pressures 20 points above normal and at risk for serious injury from falling if he forces them into meeting the guideline criteria. Guidelines are important and useful, but are just that…guidelines.

Geriatricians present what could be seen as contradictory information about medicating the elderly. On one hand, they stress the need to keep the number of medications an older adult is taking to a minimum. On the other hand, they also state that the elderly should receive the same interventions as a younger adult. Many medication recommendations for the older adult are not yet what is called evidence base practice—practice that is supported by clinical research. This is because so few studies focus on the elderly. Most research studies use younger people for their subjects. Again, guidelines are important but the clinical judgment of an experienced physician is even more important.

A second related issue is the concern over polypharmacy—multiple medications. Because many older adults have long standing chronic health problems, they may see a battery of physicians, all who are prescribing medications for the specific

74

problem they are treating. Although every doctor should be aware of all the medications a patient is taking (including over the counter medications and herbal treatments), the fragmentation of care can lead to breakdown in communications. One patient with a seizure disorder developed dilantin toxicity because she was taking dilantin capsules and phenytoin capsules, thinking they were two different medications. Dilantin is the brand name for phenytoin. Two doctors ordered it using alternate names and no one explained this to the patient who was taking double the desired dose.

Some estimate that up to 30% of the patients who come for a dementia work-up have a pseudodementia related to the combination of medications they are taking. Many may also experience a pseudodepression related to their medications. A thorough workup for dementia and depression in the elderly must include the possibility that these are side effects of their medications. In most cases decreasing the number and the dosages of the medications improved the patients' conditions remarkably.

Medications that can cause or mimic depression or dementia include:
- Beta-blockers used for hypertension such as atenolol (Tenormin), carvedilol (Coreg), metoprolol, propranolol (Inderal), sotalol

- Corticosteroids used to open airways in COPD and for inflammatory processes such as cortisone, methylprednisolone (Medrol), and prednisone
- Benzodiazepine used to reduce anxiety and to treat insomnia such as alprazolam (Xanax), diazepam (Valium), lorazepam (Ativan), temazepam (Restoril) and triazolam (Halcion). These medications can cause a paradoxical agitation in the elderly
- Also some medications for Parkinson's Disease, anticonvulsants, and hormone replacement drugs

Many medications can have synergistic effects in which a combination of drugs may greatly increase the effects of another drug (such as 1 + 1 = 3). This can lead to unwanted side effects or too much of the therapeutic effect such as dropping the blood pressure too low. Conversely, medications may hamper the effects of another medication such as vitamin K decreasing the anticoagulation (blood thinning)effect of warfarin (Coumadin).

Too often when they go to the physician with a complaint, patients and their families want to leave the doctor's office with a prescription. They feel the visit was not successful unless a medication for their complaint was prescribed. Some doctors find it easier to prescribe something for the symptom than to look further into its cause (which

76

may be a side effect of a prescribed, over the counter medicine or a home remedy) or to take time to reassure the patient that the symptoms will pass. Sam still has very mixed results in convincing people who obviously have colds that antibiotics not only will not help but can create a host of other problems (nausea, diarrhea, resistant organisms, and opportunistic infections which a healthy/untreated person would not get). If their cold has not abated in three days, they want medication. Their experience has been that if they take the antibiotics their cold will improve in a few days. Of course, in most cases it would have on its own.

Jane's father could have been the poster person for "More is Not Always Better." He complained to us that he was feeling groggy and had stumbled and fallen a couple of times. We asked for a list of his current medications and were surprised to see how many he was taking--22 in all. One of the medications he was taking was Compazine (prochlorperazine) for nausea which has the side effect of causing significant sedation. None of his physicians questioned why he was nauseated all the time or whether giving an elderly man an ongoing prescription for Compazine was appropriate. We found that another medication which he was taking for his heart failure, digoxin, was in the toxic range. Gastrointestinal disturbances are common symptoms of excessive digoxin and very old persons can develop unwanted side effects even when the medicine dose is in the "so-called," normal range. Once his digoxin dose was cut, his nausea disappeared and so did that groggy feeling and the falling since he was no longer taking the anti-nausea medication. This was a wake up call for us and we went over the list of medications carefully with him. In a few months we were able to reduce the number of medications he was taking by half without any negative effects to his overall health. Actually it was improved.

Jane's father was also diagnosed with prostate cancer in his late 70's. Prostate cancer is usually a very different and much less aggressive disease in the older male than in the middle aged male. The large majority of men over age 70 have some cancerous cells in their prostate glands but they do not die from prostate cancer. In the past most did not even learn they had prostate cancer. With the development of PSA (prostate-specific antigen) screening, 90% of prostate cancers are detected before there are symptoms. This would be good for aggressive cancers but the test does not differentiate between the slow growing and invasive types of tumors. Most men in their 70's and older would be best served through active surveillance with frequent PSA levels and tumor biopsies. The goal is to minimize causing health problems (erectile dysfunction, urinary dysfunction) in an asymptomatic man.

When Jane's father asked us whether he should take radiation treatments for his prostate cancer, we both said no. We felt the risk versus benefits were not in his favor. The treatment was more likely to do significant damage than the disease. However, the word cancer is very scary and Jane's father wanted to do "something" rather than "nothing." So he had a series of radiation treatments. The cancer was never a problem. The hemorrhagic cystitis (bleeding from the bladder) he had for the rest of his life was. The reoccurring bleeding episodes required transfusions (in one instance 8 units of blood were needed) and trips to the hospital when clots blocked his ability to urinate. Painful bladder spasms were another symptom that caused great distress. Yet we are still not sure if Jane's father knew what complications would lie ahead whether he would have chosen any differently because his fear of cancer was so great. This occurred more than a decade ago and there has been advances made in radiation treatments to minimize complications. As with all treatments, the benefits, risks, and alternatives for each individual need to be carefully explored.

One time Jane's father went into the hospital, walking on his own power, for a transfusion. He was supposed to stay overnight for monitoring of his heart failure while the blood was given. His primary doctor convinced him to stay an extra day and get some tests done to save the inconvenience of doing them as an outpatient. After visiting hours on the evening before he was to go home, a cardiologist who was covering for Jane's father's cardiologist came in and convinced him that he should have a cardiac catherization (insertion of a catheter into an artery in the leg that is then advanced to heart where dye is injected to check for cardiac blood vessel blockages and cardiac functioning.) Jane's father had great respect for doctors and never wanted to contradict those providing his care. Although Jane's father had no change in his health status at all, the cardiologist performed the catherization the next morning. The cardiologist did this without consulting Jane's father's primary physician (who knew we were all against invasive tests that would provide mostly useless information) or encouraging Jane's father to talk things over with his family.

When Jane's mother arrived the next morning she was shocked to see her husband's bed empty and stripped down. She feared the worst and was glad to know he was still alive and in the intensive care unit. He barely made it through the catherization, had a bout of kidney failure caused by the dye used in the procedure, and never walked independently again.

Despite the devastating effects of the catherization on Jane's father, a cardiac surgeon visited him in the ICU to discuss open heart surgery (which is a life saving treatment in many cases but could not really address the heart failure which was Jane's father's major problem.) In any case, the catherization did not generate any new information about his heart condition beyond that previously obtained from less invasive tests. There were no changes to be made in his treatment based on the results. Jane's father died about six weeks after having the catherization never regaining the ground that he lost. It is interesting to note that the hospital where he was treated had a fledgling open heart surgery program.

Now the question should be raised, "Where were the voices of experience when all this was going on?" A variety of factors interfered with or limited our ability to provide input into our parents' decision making about health care. We are their children and no matter how much they take pride in our accomplishments, we are not seen in the same light as the physicians they see professionally. There was also a piece of the "I don't want to be a burden" issue. (See that section.) They viewed us as being busy with careers and family and did not want to add to our obligations. They also wanted to maintain more autonomy and privacy. They knew we had opinions about their health care and sometimes they just did not want to hear or deal with them. Distance played an additional part. It is hard to stay on top of matters from a distance and we could have done this better. Finally, we did not really want to look at the fact our parents' health was failing.

In the frail elderly, more is often not better. Even the risks of diagnostic tests may outweigh their benefit. The urge to do "something" is often hard to suppress. Therefore, it is especially important to gather as much information about the risks, benefits, and alternatives for all tests and interventions. Be mindful of the elder's condition and likely prognosis (see section "Looking at the Big Picture, Am I too Old for This?") and not rush into decision making whenever possible.

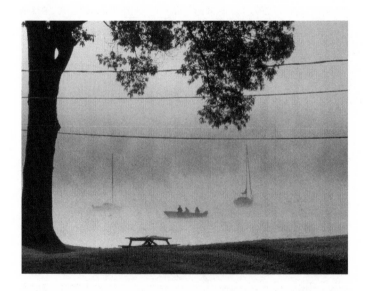

"Just to Be Sure"

The road to health care induced injury is usually paved with good intentions. The unintended consequences of unnecessary tests and treatments can be quite unpredictable and severe. An example of this is Janet Wilson. Mrs. Wilson was a spry eighty-eight year old assisted living resident. She was always up early and eager for breakfast which was her favorite meal, "Because it's hard to make a bad breakfast." She was much loved by the staff for her outgoing and upbeat attitude. She participated fully in the activities offered and looked forward to each day. One evening she was out late attending her grandson's wedding where she ate more than usual and had a glass of champagne for toasting the newlyweds.

The next morning, for the first time in memory, the staff had to wake Mrs. Wilson for breakfast. The staff were concerned that she seemed a little sluggish and to allay their fears, Mrs. Wilson made sure to eat a really good breakfast. When she stood up at the end of the meal she felt faint and unsteady. The staff rapidly intervened to prevent her from falling as she almost passed out. After a minute of sitting in the chair she was awake, alert, and embarrassed. "I guess I must have eaten too much and got up too quickly," she said. The staff had already called 911 and although her vital signs were normal and she was looking much better by the time the emergency team arrived, the staff convinced Mrs. Wilson to go to the emergency department to be checked over, "Just to be sure." Mrs. Wilson was reluctant to go but a telephone call from her niece asking her to go and get checked out made her acquiesce.

Mrs. Wilson's work up in the emergency department of the local community hospital could not identify any specific cause to her brief fainting episode. A routine urinalysis revealed some bacteria in her urine. The emergency room physician questioned her for signs and symptoms of a urinary tract infection such as burning and frequency but Mrs. Wilson did not have any of them. However, the ED physician immediately administered antibiotics and told her she would be admitted and given a course of IV antibiotics, "Just to be sure." By the time Sam was contacted, she had already received several doses in a course of the antibiotics which he would not have started.

Unfortunately, Mrs. Wilson had to wait over 36 hours in the emergency department before a bed was available. The antibiotic was making her nauseous and her appetite was poor. By the second day in the hospital being treated with antibiotics, Mrs. Wilson developed severe diarrhea. She became confused and agitated and the staff restrained her to keep her from pulling out the IV line needed for to give fluids and the antibiotics. The medications had allowed a superinfection of Clostridium difficile to take over the normal flora of bacteria in her bowel and cause colitis, an inflammation of the colon.

C. difficile is a bacterium that infects 13 in 1000 inpatients in the United States every year. It is a common bacteria that produces spores that are very hard to kill, but the good news is that C. difficile usually does not infect healthy people. Most of the people who get C. difficile are older adults who have been hospitalized and given antibiotics. The antibiotics suppress the normal protective bacteria in the gastrointestinal tract which then allows the C. difficile to flourish. The bacteria produce toxins that are irritating to the lining of the bowels.

The different type of antibiotics used to treat the C. difficile did not work for Mrs. Wilson and there was a real risk that her bowel could rupture. This would spill the infected material throughout her abdominal cavity and could be fatal. After over two weeks in the hospital, Mrs. Wilson was taken to the operating room and had her entire colon removed. She spent two weeks in intensive care and five more weeks in the hospital before being transferred to a rehabilitation facility to learn how to care for her collection bag. At this point she could barely stand. After four weeks she could walk slowly with the help of a walker. Her physical therapist thought this would probably be her new baseline and she was discharged a much changed woman back to her nursing home.

The reason Mrs. Wilson fainted was probably what she described—she ate too much and stood up too fast. It was coupled by an unusually late night the evening before and a little alcohol that might have caused some mild dehydration. She had a single episode of orthostatic hypotension(drop in blood pressure when standing) after eating. Sending her to emergency department rather than observing her more closely for the day seemed prudent but it set off a horrible chain of events.

Many women Mrs. Wilson's age are colonized by bacteria in their urinary tract. The bacteria live there but do not cause an infection. Giving her the antibiotic may have seemed prudent but it actually caused great harm. Geriatricians often need to remind other physicians to take more conservative approaches in treatment with the elderly. We wonder what would have happened if they just watched her after that first fainting spell.

"I'll Never Put Her in a Nursing Home."

A friend of ours was an only child of a single parent. Her mother was an energetic talented woman who worked into her seventies. Her mother had always been a great support providing babysitting, helping with cooking, housework, and carpooling. Our friend made sure the house she bought had a bedroom and bath for her mother. Even into her late seventies, her mother would not sit still needing to be useful, always helping with something—laundry, gardening, cooking. She was a tremendous asset to my friend and all those around her.

Somewhere around her eightieth year, our friend noticed changes in her mother's ability to function. Her cooking deteriorated to the point she served raw meat one evening. She often forgot how to do things like operate the microwave or dishwasher. She became more emotional, anxious, angry, and defensive if a problem occurred because of her declining abilities. She would confabulate (filling in lapses in memory with inappropriate information) so that my friend was not sure what actually happened to her mother while she was left alone. She started hoarding items, including food, in her room where it would rot. Finally her hygiene level became a problem. Whenever our friend would try to assist her mother with bathing, her mother would become angry and deny needing help.

She would accuse our friend of wanting to put her in a nursing home to get rid of her. Her daughter reassured her that this would never happen. Our friend told us, "I would never put her in a nursing home." We replied, "Never say 'never' and box yourself in emotionally. You don't know what the future will hold."

Things continued downhill. A daytime aide was hired to supervise our friend's mother while our friend was at work. Her mother resented the aide and the aide found it difficult to intervene and prevent unsafe behaviors. Medications to help decrease her agitation and improve her mental functioning were minimally effective. Yet our friend said, "How can I tell her she is going into a nursing home? How will I even get her in the car to go?"

Eventually it escalated to a day when our friend's mother became very agitated and began damaging the house. The aide could not stop her and called the emergency squad. She was admitted to the hospital for a change in mental status. This was a blessing in disguise as it solved the problem of moving her mother and placing her in a nursing home as she was discharged from the hospital to long term care.

After a short period of adjustment, our friend's mother initially did well in the nursing home. She responded well to the structure and activities by being less agitated and engaging with others. Later a series of small strokes caused a steep decline in her health. Her daughter visited regularly even though her mother no longer recognized her. Our friend no longer dreads coming home from work and her level of stress is greatly decreased. Yet although she knows her mother is comfortable and well cared for in the facility, she still feels guilty about not being able to keep her mother at home.

The point of this story is to keep an open mind about options. The ability each of us has to deal with stress and provide care has limits. It is often hard to imagine (or predict) what the future will bring.

Situations like this are common and making promises to yourself or others about what will be done just adds more pressure and creates more guilt. The best thing to say is that we have goals but will deal with each situation as it arises. This is one reason a living will which states health care preferences before events have occurred is not as responsive to actual situations as the health care proxy advanced directive. (See "If I Don't Discuss It, I Won't Die.")

Section Three: Quality of Life

"This Is My First Hospice Patient."

Not too long ago Sam was caring for an elderly man who did not have an obviously terminal diagnosis such as metastatic cancer but because of continuing cardiac and neurological problems was experiencing a severe decline in the quality of his life. After exploring a variety of treatment options with him and his family, it was decided at this point hospice would promote the best quality of life for him and support for his family. As part of Sam's responsibilities at the hospital where he is on staff, Sam helps supervise the residents who are building on their medical school education to become independent practitioners. The resident assigned to this man was near the end of her third and final year of residency. As Sam explained what was going on and what steps needed to be taken to place the patient on the hospice service, the resident got very excited. She stated, "This is my first hospice patient." Sam replied, "No, this is the first hospice patient you cared for who actually got hospice care."

This resident would have completed her training and started out in practice without ever having any involvement with hospice. Probably many residents have missed that opportunity. Therefore, in their future careers, hospice care is not something they are going to initially consider when planning treatment options. Hospice and palliative care will be viewed as maybe something to do when all else has been tried and failed and the person is within a few days of dying.

The purpose in telling this story is to caution you that although hospice may be a reasonable treatment option (or even the best), your health care providers may not even think about it for your loved one. You may need to present the idea of hospice care to them. In fact, they may resent your suggesting it, seeing it as a lack of faith in their abilities as the following story illustrates.

A friend of ours had an uncle in his late seventies who had several debilitating health problems that prevented him from leaving his house. He had been treated for cancer for over five years without ever going into complete remission. Complications from the chemotherapy and radiation included severe bouts of vomiting and repeated infections. He was also experiencing a decline in his mental capacities. When his niece approached the oncologist about the possibility of hospice to help coordinate her uncle's complex care and increase his comfort, the oncologist became angry and defensive. He stated that he had kept her uncle alive for five years and would keep him alive for five more. There was no discussion about the quality of her uncle's life, his diminishing abilities or what were his values and goals. The physician seemed to see the request for hospice as a lack of trust in his skills and a lack of appreciation for the care he had provided over the previous few years.

Once a patient is placed in hospice, the physician no longer has complete control of this patient's care and few people like to give up control. If my friend's mother went into hospice, the chemotherapy treatments would end.

To be balanced, many oncologists will instigate a discussion about hospice and often participate in the care of their patients at this important time. We offer this story for those who face a conflict with a particular physician. In a case like this, you may need to do more than put the idea of hospice on the table. You may need to bring in a second opinion or change physicians which is not a comfortable thing to do.

To prevent this, it is necessary to choose a physician after a frank discussion about goals and quality of life issues. Questions such as, "What is your experience with palliative care and hospice? How do you feel about DNR orders or declining interventions such as a feeding tube?"

Hospice care is a type of care which can be provided in many settings including homes, nursing homes, and inpatient units. Patients and their caregivers should assess which situation would best meets the needs.   Would the elder be more comfortable at home?

When Sam's mother was dying from a rare form of cancer, the teaching research hospital where she received her care chose her to be the first patient to receive a new experimental treatment.   The chemotherapy was photodynamic (activated only when exposed to light.) This had the advantage of limiting systemic (over all the body) side effects. The downside was it also meant she had to avoid sunlight and fluorescent lighting.   The day came when they were going to perform the procedure to activate the chemotherapy. There had to be over 15 people—students, residents, fellows, attending physicians, nurses, and technicians. For them it was a technological innovation that took the focus off the patient.   They even served cookies and water just a few feet from Sam's mother who had been without any intake for 14 hours.

The procedure was difficult for her and caused severe esophagitis (inflammation of her esophagus) making swallowing food impossible. Eventually she needed a feeding tube placed into her stomach.   Again, the medical staff was very willing to do this.   Within a short time, however, she decided, "It was no longer worth it," and she went into hospice. This was an option the treatment team never discussed with her but she was familiar with it because she utilized hospice services with Sam's father.

Once she went into hospice we never heard from anyone at the teaching research hospital again. She died a few weeks later, cared for by the two aides who had cared for Sam's father when he was dying from Alzheimer's Disease. They knew her, loved her, and she felt comfort in their care. As for the teaching research hospital, we ask ourselves, "What are they actually teaching the students, residents and fellows about caring for people?"

Hospice care is one part of the continuum of care that is called palliative. The goal of palliative care is to provide relief from negative symptoms such as pain, nausea, or shortness of breath, without trying to cure the underlying disease process. A person does not have to be at the end of life and in hospice to be a good candidate for palliative care. Having any chronic illness that is causing debilitating symptoms would make someone suitable for palliative care. It does not mean curative treatment cannot be pursued at the same time. Palliative care can be an adjunct to it. Providing care whose only goal is to make the patient more comfortable would seem to be noncontroversial. Yet we have heard physicians speak very disparagingly about palliative care to the point that some physicians refused to allow any mention of it when discussing their patients.

Studies have shown that until recently there has been very little emphasis on palliative and hospice care in medical school and training. In the past, clinical practice guidelines for chronic diseases that would benefit greatly from palliation were limited. The focus was on acute curative care even for conditions that were not curable. This has changed and many hospitals now have palliative care experts on staff, but some physicians still will not utilize their services for their patients. Again you need to find out what perspective your physician has regarding palliative care and hospice. You do not want to limit you treatment choices.

Studies have shown that many people enter hospice too late to take advantage of all its services such as nursing and home health aide care, psychological and spiritual counseling, and respite care. They wait until death is imminent—within a week or less—before considering hospice. (See "Hospice? I'm Not Ready to Give up.")

"Hospice? I'm Not Ready to Give Up."

One of the greatest misconceptions about hospice care is that it means "giving up." Whenever we introduce hospice into the discussion of treatment options, families and even patients (though patients less so) immediately reject the possibility of entering hospice because it seems too negative and defeatist. They are not ready to "throw in the towel" and give up the fight. Many physicians and other health care workers also have this attitude. This is unfortunate because hospice is not the absence of therapy. It has a wealth of resources to offer patients and their families that would probably meet their needs more satisfactorily than continued acute interventions. All of our parents were in hospice care when they died (from over 6 months to one day). Three died at home and one in a nursing home with a hospice facility.

A metaphor for understanding this could be the experience of driving to a cabin in the woods. At first you are driving down the highway in a high-powered sports car. You can go fast. It feels good. But by the end of the trip the road becomes rough and uneven. Staying in the sports car will not get you where you want to go and may even cause an accident. Switching to a less glamorous sport utility vehicle (SUV) makes more sense and will get you where you want to go. Driving an SUV is not giving up on driving altogether. It is a practical response to the change in the road. Switching to hospice care is not giving up on providing care. It is a practical response to the change in the patient's status and providing the care that is now needed.

Of course it does mean coming to grips with a very sad reality. "We're going to help Mom have the most comfortable end of life experience possible," Sam said as he sat by the bedside of a 95 year old woman, Eleanor Breed, with her son. He was setting the stage for a discussion of hospice. The patient had been a dynamo. She was a college graduate. No small feat for a woman of her generation. Eleanor had served as a captain in the WACs and then ran a successful real estate business with her husband of fifty years. Her son began almost every conversation about his mother with a brief recitation of her accomplishments. This preamble allowed him to go on with the rest uncomfortable discussion that was to follow..

His mother had lived independently until about six months ago when she had hip replacement surgery. This current admission from a rehabilitation facility was because she had developed pneumonia. The blood vessels to her legs were malfunctioning and she had developed gangrene of one of her toes. The vascular doctors (blood vessel specialists) did not feel she would do well with a bypass operation on the clogged blood vessels and recommended that the entire foot be amputated. In addition she was becoming so weak that she could not even swallow properly. Sam and the son reviewed all of these issues as they sat quietly looking at his mother. "Who was he seeing?" Sam wondered, "The mother of his youth or the woman she is now?"

Sam began addressing each issue and what could be done including the insertion of the feeding tube. The son realized his hope that aggressive care might get the mother he remembered back was unrealistic. Sam explained that such an outcome, even under the best of circumstances, was extremely unlikely, and that the various treatments were guaranteed to cause significant pain and suffering. The son had already seen the need for both physical and chemical restraint in order to prevent his mother from removing her intravenous lines and other catheters. He admitted that she would not want to be alive under such circumstances unless she could resume her independent life. Sam assured him that the chances of her living independently were, in his experience, zero.

You might ask how can anyone be so sure and are we always right? The answer does not come out of arrogance or any special feeling of superiority. In some ways, it is sad and difficult to have to be the one to deliver such news. When one has seen situations such as the one we have described above and when none have ever resumed a life they would ever want to have, one can bring this level of certainty to families struggling to make difficult decisions. Over several days, he came to the conclusion that the hospice approach was right for his mother and plans were made to implement his decision.

Hospice can help patients and their families use the time remaining most effectively to resolve old grievances and strengthen relationships. The patient receiving palliative care is more comfortable and able to interact more fully. Providing support and care at the end-of-life can be rewarding to friends and family. One friend gathered her family around and they sang to her husband as he died. This is not giving up. This is consciously choosing a different path.

One more story to emphasize the point that choosing hospice is not giving up. Mrs. Patricia Reynolds was a woman in her 90's with metastatic (wide spread) breast cancer. She lived alone and had few social resources. Mrs. Reynolds was rapidly failing because of multiple health problems. Her appetite was poor. She had chronic pain which interfered with her sleep; she was lonely and depressed. The quality of her life was very poor and her life expectancy was short. She agreed to have home hospice. With proper analgesia her pain was much better managed and her appetite and sleeping improved. She had more energy and her interest in life returned. Having the social support services of hospice reduced her loneliness. The decline in her health status continued but at a much slower pace because her basic needs for nutrition, sleep, comfort and socialization were being met. These issues are often better addressed in hospice than acute care. She died after two years in hospice. She probably lived much longer in hospice than she would have lived without hospice care and during the two years had a much better quality of life.

This brings up another misconception about hospice—that the patient must have six months or less to live. The time frame of six months comes from Medicare reimbursement guidelines. However, there is awareness that determining a life expectancy is imperfect as there are so many variables that intervene. The expectation in hospice is that the person has a life limiting illness with about a six month life expectancy if the disease process takes its normal course. Unfortunately, too many people wait until death is imminent and therefore the advantages of hospice care are not as fully utilized. (See "This is My First Hospice Patient")

Older adults tend to be referred to hospice earlier than other age groups. There is a trend for frail elderly with multiple chronic health problems who are in decline to choose hospice care toward the end of their lives. This speaks to another misconception about hospice—that it is only for people with cancer. Although cancer is the most common diagnosis in hospice patients, congestive heart failure, chronic obstructive airway disease, Alzheimer's Disease, failure to thrive, and cerebral vascular accidents (CVA, stroke), are common diagnoses.

As mentioned earlier, patients may be more open to the idea of hospice than their families, but they may not bring the topic up because their families keep telling them to "fight." While encouraging the "good fight" is well intentioned, it sometimes comes across as condemning. If the patient does not get better, it is as if the patient is not fighting hard enough. Some people may have had cancer and say, "I fought it and won and so can you." They may not know that every disease has a range of severity and their experience will not necessarily be the same as another's. Also, the older we get, the more likely we are to have other underlying health problems that may make "fighting" more difficult.

Families may not bring up the topic of hospice for fear that the patient will feel abandoned. Both patients and families may ignore or reject hospice because neither want to acknowledge to the other than there is an end approaching. They are keeping up a "good front" at the expense of honest talk and beneficial decision making.   As the patient's health fails, it takes more and more effort by everyone to deny what is going on.   The discomfort in maintaining the pretense diminishes the opportunity to say meaningful good-byes.

On the other side of the equation are the people who choose hospice and are impatient to die. Both our mothers chose hospice (one for cancer; one for heart failure).   Both were extremely unhappy with their health status and their poor quality of life. Both had very limited life expectancies (months). They felt they had led good lives but were now ready to end their suffering. There were no further treatments for Sam's mother's cancer and the option of open heart surgery was rejected by Jane's mother because of the decline in so many other areas of health (vision, hearing, memory). "I don't want to have a fixed heart and sit around for years blind and deaf. Besides I've had open heart surgery before and I don't want to go through it again"

Both women had the misconception that once they entered hospice they could relax and die quickly—that hospice equaled death. When Jane's mother entered inpatient hospice, she told every staff member who entered the room in a cheerful voice, "I've had a good life. I'm ready to go." Sam's mother decided continuing aggressive cancer treatment was no longer worth it. (See section, "Is it Worth it?") Both were disappointed when they spent 2 to 8 weeks in hospice. Fortunately, the supportive care they received through hospice made that time as comfortable as possible.

We recommend that people who are uncertain about hospice get second opinions and learn about the most advanced therapies for their disease. There are many fine complementary therapies (also called alternative therapies) such as acupuncture and biofeedback that have been shown to relieve discomfort and improve the quality of life. Be careful, however, of unverified treatments offered by people outside of the mainstream medical establishment. There are charlatans who prey on the vulnerability of terminal patients, offering expensive, useless, and even dangerous treatments. We have seen unfortunate people with treatable cancers who chose unproven therapies that wasted their time and money. By the time they came back to conventional proven treatment, they could no longer be cured.

For family members, knowing all reasonable options have been considered helps to relieve guilt over "not doing enough." There may be options besides hospice that will better meet the patient's needs initially. The best example of this is a friend who had been treated for cancer at a fine local teaching hospital and relapsed again. The oncologists told him there was nothing more they could do and recommended hospice. He was told he would probably live at most another six months. Our friend said, "I'm not ready to give up," and went to a well-known cancer institution and began a new chemotherapy protocol. Although the treatments were very difficult, they gave him over two more years of quality living before he died. He never used hospice care but felt fully supported by the staff at the hospital where he had been receiving care for his last two years.

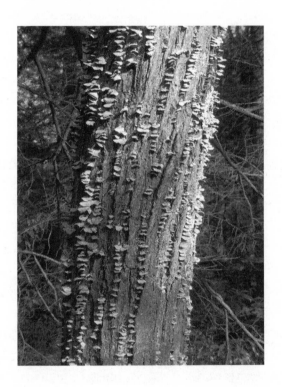

"I Don't Want to Be a Burden."

Boyd Moss was a widower in his mid-80's when he came to see Sam for a variety of mild to moderate chronic health problems.   As Sam was soon to learn, Mr. Moss had always been an impatient and demanding person.   His wife had served as a buffer through the years, but with her death, his difficult personality became more of an issue. After the initial visit, Mr. Moss would show up in Sam's office without an appointment and get angry if he could not be seen quickly despite seeing that there were people in the waiting room.   When Sam became concerned about a growing health issue, he asked Mr. Moss for permission to call one of his children.   Mr. Moss replied, "I don't want to be a burden."   He added, "Besides, they never bother with me, so don't waste your time."

After some coaxing, Mr. Moss finally agreed to let Sam speak with his daughter who lived locally.   Sam was surprised to find that she was very concerned about her father's welfare, called him every day, and stopped by with food twice a week.   When Sam tried to reconcile this with Mr. Moss's statement about their lack of interest, Mr. Moss stated, "They aren't a help. They don't live with me."   Anything less than living with him (or perhaps asking him to live with them) meant his family did not want to be bothered by him. The underlying message is "If you don't do exactly as I want, then you really don't want to be a help. You think I am a burden."

The expression, "I don't want to be a burden," is another phrase Jane discusses in her "Keeping Emotionally Fit as We Age" lecture. What does it really mean? "I don't want to be a burden," can mean exactly what it says. The elder may realize that family members are busy with their own lives and does not want to add to their load. We have all heard of the "Sandwich Generation," those middle aged adults still parenting their growing children while assuming more and more of the care of their own parents. Older adults may not ask for help and hope that the problem will resolve on its own without burdening their adult children. They may be keenly aware of their adult children's limitations—emotionally, financially, and physically. They do not want to cause guilty feelings by asking more of their children than their children can provide. The older adults may prefer to have a diminished quality of life rather than negatively impact (in their perception) their children's lives.

However, as Sam tells his patients, "If you need assistance and refuse help, especially in areas related to safety issues, rather than not being a burden, you create more stress for those caring for you." If the elder with balance problems refuses to use a cane or wear a fall alert pendant, every time a child (or other responsible person) calls and no one answers, there will be anxiety—"Have they fallen? Are they hurt?" By not keeping family and friends abreast of the current situation and taking appropriate help but instead saying, "I don't want to be a burden," the elder denies or ignores the legitimate concerns of loved ones.   Instead of being able to put into place help that will keep the elder safe and improve the quality of life, the child dreads every telephone call.

"I don't want to be a burden," can also express a desire to maintain control and privacy. Most people want to live independently and make their own choices for good or for bad. They do not want someone looking over their shoulder second guessing them. Why should it be any different as we age?   The older adult may be willing to trade some quality of life for the ability to be independent. The elderly may correctly anticipate that if someone else looks into their situation, their privacy may be sacrificed by the introduction of supportive personnel into their home or, worse yet, the move to assisted living or some other less private residential setting.

Individuals have a wide range of needs for socialization.   Some prefer more solitary time. They can be alone without being lonely.   "I don't want to be a burden," can just be an extension of the desire to have more "personal space." Daily telephone calls and frequent visits may be seen more as intrusions than welcomed signs of caring. It is not that they do not want to be a burden, it is they do not want to be bothered by others.

Some people say, "I don't want to be a burden," because they secretly fear they will be hurt if their requests for help are disregard. They would rather muddle on by themselves and never have to face the possibility of being ignored or rejected. Perhaps, they have already made some simple requests and met with indifference or, worse, hostility.

In a few unfortunate cases, "They never bother with me," is an accurate statement. Sam has seen families that have shown little interest in their elder until death is near. Is it a reflection of past abusive or dysfunctional family relationships? Elder neglect and abuse is seen more often in families that have previously known partner and child abuse.

In some cases, family members suddenly materialize expressing concern. Did the elder's condition need to get to this critical point to get their attention? Do they want to try to work things out one last time? Are they motivated by guilt or greed? Family dynamics are extremely complex.

Mr. Moss's comment, "They never bother with me," was incorrect. As stated earlier, it may be that because he did not get the exact care he wanted, he felt neglected. Caring for a person like him is emotionally draining.

Some people are unable to acknowledge the help of others and by saying "Thank you." They will try to use guilt to get what they want and are never satisfied. A caregiver in this situation needs to assess the situation realistically (not colored by the elder's manipulation) and determine what support can be provided. Limit setting is critical as is knowing your own limits. Acknowledge the difficulty of the situation. Accept the elder's weaknesses and not seek the emotional support that will never be given. Otherwise, caregiver burnout is likely to arise.

Signs of caregiver burnout include sadness or depression (loss of appetite or overeating, difficulty sleeping, poor concentration, inability to enjoy life), decreased overall physical health (frequent infections, general malaise, lack of energy, pain), feeling overwhelmed (want to give up, do not know what else to do, never feeling satisfied with performance).

Ways to prevent or recover from caregiver burnout include:

- Keep the elder's circle of family and friends informed about the situation and the level of care being provided
- Share responsibilities with other family members and paid help.
- Set aside time each day to relax (prayer, meditation, warm bath, deep breathing)
- Do an enjoyable activity daily (read, listen to music, walk the dog)
- Assume additional responsibilities (work, volunteer civic groups) cautiously
- Find a safe outlet to express your feelings (close friend, journal, clergy, counselor, support group, art)
- Pay attention to your health (exercise regularly, eat healthy, keep regular sleep schedule)
- Set aside worry times (15 minutes each morning and evening) and not allow yourself to worry at other times
- Review your expectations and how you talk to yourself. Be careful not to berate yourself because you cannot make others happy.
- Do not be afraid to ask for help.
- Do not be afraid to say "no" (or at least, "not at this time.")

"Is It Worth It?"

The question "Is it worth it? "gets to the crux of the issue of longevity versus quality of life. This often occurs when a person with a poor prognosis is facing grueling treatments. Most people are willing to sacrifice a short term loss in quality of life for a chance at a much longer life. The variables of how much more life they can buy and at what cost are the critical issues. As we get closer to the end of our life expectancy, how we balance longevity versus quality of life usually changes.

As we have already mentioned, predicting how much longer someone with a terminal illness (not just cancer but processes such as end stage heart disease) is difficult. Physicians often overestimate the time remaining to offer patients and family hope.

On the other hand, we all know people who were given "months to live" and who are still with us years later. This does not mean the disease process was cured. It usually means the progression of the disease slowed more than anticipated or they received new treatments or made lifestyle modifications that were effective.

The decision about what losses and side effects are acceptable is very individual. Changes that would have been deemed intolerable early in the decline of health may become acceptable as the disease progresses.

Jane had a friend, John, with severe COPD (Chronic Obstructive Pulmonary Disease). He was an active man both professionally and socially with a large extended family. When first diagnosed, he mostly had to pace his activities to prevent shortness of breath. He would say to Jane, "If I ever become oxygen dependent, I would rather be dead." When the time came that he needed continuous oxygen, John learned to live with it. In fact, he became the master of portable oxygen, BiPap machines (which provide positive airway pressure to assist breathing), and a host of other technologies and techniques to support his diminishing respiratory function. His ability to utilize assistive technologies allowed him to get out and around and stay connected. The steroid medications he used to keep his airways open caused a host of side effects. John learned how to minimize the side effects and live with those he could not avoid. Until the very last days of his life, John was as active and connected as he could be despite the limitations of his condition. He never stopped trying to find another way of getting a little more time.

Sam's mother who had the rare bile duct cancer being treated with photodynamic therapy

(See "This is My First Hospice Patient") made different choices. One day she asked Jane, "Is it worth it?" Jane replied, "When it is no longer worth it, you won't have to ask." Although the physicians did not offer any hope for a cure, they thought this new experimental treatment could "buy" her more time. She endured a tremendous amount of pain and disability without complaint. Despite the toll on her quality of life, she was willing to pay the price for the possibility of living longer. When complications caused changes that required more personally invasive treatment, she decided it was no longer worth it. She had reached the tipping point between quality of life and longevity. She went into hospice the next day, stopped all treatments and medications, and died in just over a week.

The point of both these stories is to realize that the answer to "Is it worth It?" is hard to predict and will probably change over time. Just as we cautioned in the story "I will Never Put Her in a Nursing Home," keep your mind and options open. If you are not sure about an intervention or treatment, you can start it and give yourself permission to stop when you want. This is true of most interventions such as radiation, medications, and chemotherapy. Obviously surgery is an all or nothing choice. Some interventions such as putting someone on a ventilator or using a feeding tube may be easier emotionally to start than discontinue.

113

There are differing religious opinions about what must be done and what can be stopped once started. If that information is important to you, consult your clergy early in the process. Again, family and friends may have conflicting thoughts about what should or should not be done. Laying a foundation with others about the choices to be made may help diminish conflict. In the end, the decision rests with the patient or health care agent.

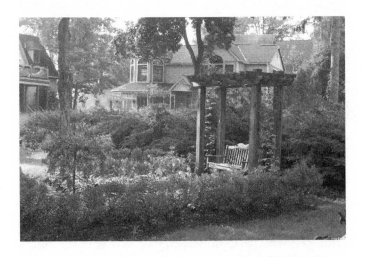

"What Would Dad Want?"

Fred Morgan had three sons, all ambitious and successful. Larry, the oldest, was a psychiatrist in California, Phil a local pharmacist, and Jack, the youngest, an attorney in Maryland. Fred, also a pharmacist, ran a five store business in Brooklyn until Phil graduated from pharmacy school and joined his dad in the business. Fred remained active in the business until he turned 82. One day he told his family, "I'm ready to slow down. Okay, I'm exhausted." None of the children, including, Phil saw this coming.

Mary was Fred's wife of 57 years. She had died of dementia three years earlier. Fred had hired a wonderful staff to be with his wife while he worked but did much of her physical care whenever he was home. He realized that Mary barely knew who he was but always said, "She likes when I help."

A year after he retired, Fred had a stroke leaving him barely able to walk and in need of 24 hour care. Only Phil, who lived nearby, was able to visit his dad frequently. Larry and Jack each alternated monthly visits to give Phil and his wife a chance to get away. Although Sam had never met Larry and Jack, the situation seemed as ideal as possible. There were enough resources to maintain Fred's physical care and the sons seemed to help each other out in a reasonable way. Sam assumed that as Fred's condition worsened, there would not be much conflict in making end of life decisions.

When Fred suddenly became unresponsive late one Friday afternoon, his home attendant, Lorinda, called 911. Sam was called by the emergency room physician and informed that Fred had pneumonia and was dehydrated. He was given intravenous fluids and antibiotics in the emergency room and was already starting to respond. Sam called Phil who said he would be there in an hour and would bring a copy of Fred's health care proxy.

About four days after admission Fred had not improved. He slept unless someone aroused him. He ate poorly. Liquid supplements were added to Fred's diet but the nutrition staff who had been monitoring his case called after a week. The nutritionist recommended initiating artificial nutrition—a feeding tube. Sam spoke to Phil whose name was first on the health care proxy, "No way. Dad said he'd never want that." Sam told Phil to have Fred's private aides encourage Fred to take more by mouth and that we'd see how things were going in a couple of days.

The next day Sam got an irate call from Larry who was visiting from Los Angeles. "Phil may be the health care agent, but I am the oldest and a physician. Dad's wasting away. He needs a feeding tube or he's going to starve to death. I will not let that happen" Of all the families Sam had dealt with over the years, this was the last one he would have expected to have this reaction. Sam had wrongly assumed that the brothers were talking to each other and that they would all abide by Fred's wishes. Sam did not wait to hear from Jack before setting up a meeting with the three brothers, late in the day in one of the hospital's conference rooms.

Each son brought a spouse and at least one child to the conference. There were twelve present. Usually having this large a number of people present complicates things. The possibility for personal agendas and interpersonal conflict escalates. After some tense opening remarks, one of the grandchildren asked, "Is Grandpa going to make it?"

This was perhaps the best and most difficult question. In treating frail (previous stroke, trouble walking, poor nutrition, poor mobility) patients like Fred, sudden severe illnesses can be life ending. Also, in most cases, patients in Fred's condition rarely return to their pre-hospitalization status. Sam replied, "He'll probably make it out of the hospital but very likely will never be as good as he was before." He then reminded the family that even before he developed pneumonia, Fred was greatly diminished from the dynamo they loved. They needed to readjust their perceptions about Fred's status.

Phil and Larry argued over artificial nutrition. Jack, Fred's attorney son, spoke dispassionately but, in his own way, with the most love. He stated that Fred's wishes should be honored. Almost all the grandchildren agreed and Fred was discharged home two days later. Hospice was called in after about a month, and Fred died in his own bed under the watchful eye of his aide, Lorinda. At the funeral, the family celebrated Fred and Mary's wonderful life.

Fred Morgan's story illustrates many important end-of-life lessons that improve the quality of life for the patient and the caregivers.

- Sharing in the care of a loved one is better for everyone. It prevents resentments among family members and increases the likelihood that their understanding of the situation is similar.
- Advanced directives make difficult decisions easier.
- Whoever is making the health care decision –the patient, the patient's agent or physician-- should always get input from key persons involved. In Fred's case, Phil and Sam should

have made sure that all of the brothers were involved in the decision about artificial nutrition.

- Do not assume that because a family member/friend is a health care professional his or her opinion is necessarily correct. Sometimes he or she can provide a better understanding of the situation. Sometimes, as in Jack's case, emotions may cloud judgment as with anyone else.

- Recognize that current decision making may be colored by family history. It may also be seen as an opportunity to establish control and power within the family dynamics.

- Accept that some friends and family will be better able to adjust to your love one's declining abilities than others. Some will offer wonderful support; others will find the situation too difficult/ painful and disappear.

- Having wonderful caregivers such as Fred's, Lorinda, is so important. Making sure that Lorinda understood the plan for Fred's care after he went home is a point not made in the story but crucial for Fred and in consideration of Lorinda's feelings. (See "Don't Call 911.")

"A Different Kind of Hope."

Richard Brown was 72 years young. He was a retired business executive who played golf three times a week at his country club. He was active in his community and he and his wife, Roberta, had a rich life together full of family, friends, and travel. One evening at dinner, he collapsed at the table. By the time the paramedics arrived and restarted his heart, he had suffered anoxic encephalopathy—brain tissue death from lack of oxygen. He lay in his hospital bed, the picture of health—fit and tanned—except for all the tubes that connected him to the machinery that was keeping him alive. The time had come to decide whether to create permanent surgical openings for these necessary tubes or to allow Mr. Brown to die.

Mr. Brown's wife and his daughter were willing to forego more aggressive interventions. The two other children, his sons, were unwilling to "give up hope." This was very understandable, especially because he looked so good-- just asleep and ready to wake up. The sons felt they were being disloyal to their father by not hoping for the best. There probably was also an unconscious piece, which we all carry in us from childhood, that wishing for something hard enough will make it happen. (Or that if we don't think positive thoughts, something bad will happen.) However, their father's condition was not ambiguous, he was not going to recover his normal mental functions and return to any level of his former self. He would stay on the ventilator with a PEG tube, immobilized and incontinent until he died perhaps months or even years later from an infection or another cardiac event.

When Jane talked with the sons, she focused on the word "hope" and what it meant. She said that hope for a complete recovery while understandable was unrealistic based on the information we had—it was not going to happen. But it could be replaced by a different kind of hope that would better serve their father. It would be the hope that their father would avoid unnecessary pain and suffering. It was the hope that their father's dignity would be maintained. It was the hope that they would remember him as the vital active man that he was and not as the unresponsive dwindling being he would become over the next weeks and months if intensive treatment was maintained. It was the hope to do what they think their father would choose for himself (if he could) facing his current condition and with his prognosis. These hopes are just as real and important as the hope for significant recovery because they are based in reality. They are hopes that can be fulfilled for the patient's welfare.

Within a day or two, the Brown family was able to reach a consensus about what to do for Mr.

121

Brown. Aggressive treatment was stopped and he died shortly thereafter. Our hope for him is that his family has been able to recall wonderful memories of him and feel that their decision to let him go in peace was the right one.

One final note—every once in a while there is an article in the paper about someone who has been in a coma for years waking up and talking. These extremely rare events are grasped by people with loved ones with severe brain injuries as reinforcement to keep intensive measures going. Without going into great neurological detail, there are various levels of unconsciousness. Not all comas are equal. Some may be temporary and last up to a month with a gradual return of functioning. Others have such physiological changes that recovery is impossible. People in a persistent vegetative state have severe brain damage. However, they will open their eyes reflexively. Family and even staff may read into this eye opening and believe the patient is responding to their words and actions. This again is a very understandable response. But almost always if an autopsy is performed, it indicates that the eye opening could not be purposeful as there was no higher brain functioning for recognition and response.

Section Four: Health Care Decision Making

"Don't Call 911."

Many older adults have come to terms with the limitations and downside of acute care treatment for their chronic illnesses and frailty. They wish to avoid going to the emergency department and being admitted to the hospital. Many wish to die at home. Despite the reasonableness of their choice and its communication to caregivers, we have found that the impulse to call 911 is hard to ignore. A family member or caregiver may get frightened by the process of dying and call 911. It is important at the that everyone who is taking care of the dying person be familiarized with what to expect and be comfortable in not reaching out for emergency care.

There may be a pre-active period of dying in which the patient feels that death is approaching and starts withdrawing from life—talking and eating less, sleeping more. The patient may make an effort to have his or her final say or be less interactive. Usually overall health will decline. Whatever is the underlying problem will get worse. This can go on for several weeks.

When patients are actively dying, they often become unresponsive or may moan and cry. Bodily functions such as urination may cease. The

123

extremities may become cold, mottled, or bluish. Alterations in breathing—periods of breathlessness—become apparent. Mucus and saliva may accumulate in the back of the throat creating a gurgling sound. It may appear that people are struggling for breath, but at this point they are at the very end and not felt to be suffering. (However, turning them on their side can help clear the airway.)

As these changes occur, those watching may become frightened and feel helpless. The urge to call for assistance can be strong. The caregivers want to do something. Measures such as mouth care, skin care, and positioning are the best interventions as they make dying patients more comfortable. This is a time to discuss with the health care provider about being liberal with pain medications such as Roxanol (liquid morphine) and anti-anxiety agents such as Ativan (lorazepam). Letting a loved one go in a supportive environment surrounded by caring people is not an easy process, but is the best last gift.

When a person is chronically, but not terminally, ill the urge to call 911 when an acute change occurs is even stronger. Sam had a patient who was in his late 80's, Dan Brickman, who had a series of small strokes (CVAs, brain attacks) that had left him with considerable physical impairment. He was lucid and being cared for at home by a wonderful team of aides. He clearly stated to everyone that he did not ever want to be re-hospitalized. One day he had another small stroke. He was going in and out of consciousness. His daughter was called by the aide and after talking with Sam decided to keep her father at home and comfortable. The daughter called her own daughter to tell her what was happening. The granddaughter wanted more information about her grandfather's condition and called 911. She did not intend to intervene in how the situation was handled and did not realize that once the 911 system is activated, it is hard to change the course of events.

When the emergency team came to Mr. Brickman's apartment, the aide was shocked to see them. Although there was a home DNR in place (the DNR from a hospitalization does not transfer to the home), it was not applicable in the current situation since he had not stopped breathing. There was a health care proxy in place for the daughter to make decisions but the emergency medical technicians did not want to be the ones to determine if Mr. Brickman lacked capacity so that they would not follow his daughter's telephone instructions. Even talking to Sam on the telephone did not dissuade them from their intention of bringing him to the hospital. (In support of the EMT's they really did not have the authority to do anything else. They were doing their job correctly.) Although he had been unable to speak all afternoon, when asked if he

125

wanted to go to the hospital, Mr. Brickman was able to say, "No." He remained at home and received supportive care. He recovered from the stroke over the next few weeks and returned to his usual state of health.

Hospitals are difficult environments for the elderly. They are more likely to experience iatrogenic illness (illnesses caused through health care) such as infections, falls, and delirium. The emergency departments (EDs) and intensive care units (ICUs) of hospitals save lives daily. They are also the most taxing hospital environment for the elderly. Most lack windows and have bright lights and noisy activity around the clock. The older adult has to contend with a sea of new faces. The equipment from the relatively simple IV pump to more complex EKG monitors can be confusing and frightening. The environment impedes anyone's ability to rest, sleep, or eat properly. This triggers further deterioration.

Many patients are forced to stay in EDs for several days awaiting a bed. Delirium (a period of agitated confusion) is a complication for people of any age in EDs and ICUs, but the elderly are particularly vulnerable. Recent research supports that repeated hospitalizations and ICU admissions at the end of life decrease quality of life.

This is why every effort should be made to keep older people out of the hospital. If hospitalization is required, it should be as brief as possible. We strongly advise having an aide or family member stay at the bedside, especially during meals.

Early mobilization is critical. The elderly should be out of bed for meals and ambulated regularly. For example, if a hip fracture which requires surgery is not operated on within 24 hours, the rate of serious complications such as pneumonia increases greatly. With the availability of many treatments at home (such as physical therapy, IV therapy, and wound care), the elderly, their family, and their physicians should explore every option before hospitalizing an older adult.

Here is a final note about the elderly who live in nursing homes. Nursing homes do not like their residents dying in their facility. They will often send patients for whom acute care has little to offer to hospitals to avoid having a death on their records. This does not mean there are not legitimate reasons to hospitalize nursing home patients. The decision to do so can come from real concern for the resident. However, if the elder or the family does not want the risks of hospitalization, they need to carefully question the purpose behind the transfer to an acute care facility. They need to be clear about their treatment choices and communicate them effectively the nursing home (or assisted living) staff and physicians.

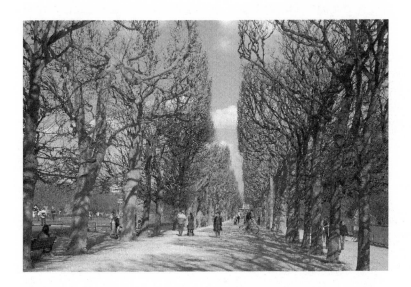

"You Don't Want Him to Die, Do You?"

Communication is a key element when making difficult decisions about health care for yourself or a loved one. When people are anxious and in a strange environment (which is the case for many patients and families in a health care setting) it is harder to hear and comprehend what is being said. The health care providers (HCPs) may feel rushed, tired, or distracted, and may not do the best job in providing information clearly. Many health care providers forget to stop talking in "medicalese". They use terminology that may be difficult for the lay person to understand. Too often people are afraid or embarrassed to ask for an explanation, but it is absolutely appropriate to ask the HCP to explain things in lay terms. This does not mean talking down to a person, but presenting the material more slowly and in more easily understood language.

Here's an example. "Why can't dad swallow?" "The xerostomia secondary to the anticholinergic effects of his medications combined with CNS malfunction in the brain stem is causing problems with deglutition leading to dysphagia thereby preventing adequate oral intake." "Doctor, could you please rephrase that? I could not understand some of your terms." "Oh. Okay. Your dad has a dry mouth possibly related to some of the medicines. Also the small stroke he had affected the part of the brain involved in swallowing. This makes it difficult for him to swallow so he's just not taking in enough."

Many times physicians underestimate the physical and emotional cost of procedures and treatments. They present the best case scenario as if it were the usual outcome. With any diagnostic procedure, one must ask the question, "Will this test change the way my loved one is treated?" Also ask, "How much suffering does this procedure entail in the short and long run?" When considering treatments, similar questions about the actual toll on the patient and realistic benefits should be asked.

As life supporting technologies multiply, the need for in-depth conversations about treatment options becomes more critical. If language and cultural differences enter into the process, discussions about the complex issues related to providing care to the older adult easily become disjointed. Jane remembers caring for an older man who came from a rural area to the burn unit where she was working. He needed to have surgery to amputate a severely infected arm. The anesthesiologist who had a very thick accent went into his room to provide informed consent. Jane observed their interaction and was concerned about what was being communicated. When she asked the patient to tell her what he understood about what the doctor said, the patient replied, "We're going somewhere together and he (the doctor) is going to sleep." The patient had not realized he was being prepared for his arm to be amputated.

The expression, "It's just semantics," is used to make the point that although the words are different they really mean the same thing. In the difficult conversations that take place during a complex illness or at the end of life, the choice of words carries emotional baggage and subtle but deep nuances. One example that makes this clear is the discussion about treatment options near the end of life. Currently most institutions use the term DNR (do not resuscitate) to eliminate performing CPR (cardiopulmonary resuscitation) on patients who are unlikely to benefit from it. Some even add the DNI (do not intubate) which means not placing a plastic tube through the mouth into the airway to support breathing.

By using the negative terms of withholding treatment, do not resuscitate or intubate, the family may feel it is choosing not to do all that could be done for their loved one. This often triggers feelings of guilt. To avoid this guilt they will not sign the DNR. There is an underlying fear that the patient will not be properly cared for if the DNR is in place. In actuality, DNR/ DNI is the only part of care to change. However, there may be some policies regarding placement in ICU's or the performing of surgical procedures if there is a DNR.

As stated in the Section Five chapter on futile care and health care decision making, current studies show that less than 20% of elderly people who receive CPR survive and get discharged from the hospital. Their dying may have been delayed by a few days or weeks but most of the patients did not recover enough to be discharged. Did this temporary delay in dying provide an opportunity for closure and closeness or did it only prolong suffering in someone unable to communicate?

CPR is a very aggressive intervention. The chest is compressed about 2 inches to force blood from the heart. Sometimes an endotracheal tube is inserted through the mouth down the airway to the lungs and taped into place. Then someone manually pumps air into the lungs. Electric shocks are delivered to try to restart the heart's rhythmic beating. Medications are pushed into the bloodstream. Complications from CPR include rib fractures, punctured collapsed lungs, and lacerated liver. When we thought about many of the very elderly population (the old old) patients we have seen receive CPR treatment in the hospital, we concluded that the percentage that has been "successfully resuscitated," must be much lower than 20%. In our experience, the frail elderly who needed multiple episodes of resuscitation never went home.

The Rev. Chuck Meyer was Vice President of Operations and Chaplain at St. David's Medical Center in Austin, Texas and an expert on health care ethics. He started a campaign to change the DNR policy to an allow-natural-death (AND) policy about fifteen years ago. The term has not become common and we believe it should be used more. The AND reflects an acceptance of death as part of life and not a failure of acute treatment. It supports the provision of comfort measures rather than pursuing an impossible cure which usually becomes a delay of death and prolonged suffering. The DNR order is only a decision to withhold one specific intervention, cardiopulmonary resuscitation.

The question, "You Don't Want Him to Die, Do You?" implies that the care being proposed will prevent the person from dying rather than delaying the dying process. One area where this can be seen in process is in the placement and removal of artificial feeding devices in patients with severe permanent brain injury and dementia.

In our opinion, one of the most misused pieces of technology has been the PEG which stands for Percutaneous (through the skin) Endoscopic (using a special instrument called an endoscope for the purpose of inserting the tube) Gastrostomy (a surgically created hole in the stomach). A plastic catheter goes through the abdominal wall into the stomach and is used to feed patients who are unable to swallow. It had been developed as a feeding device for patients who could no longer tolerate NG tubes (nasogastric tubes) which go through the nose into the stomach. Because NG tubes cause irritation to the lining of nose and throat and increase the chance of aspiration (food coming up from the stomach and going into the lung), they cannot be left in for very long. Patients who need long term nutritional support are candidates for PEG tubes. They improve the nutritional status and may hasten healing of wounds and increase general wellbeing. They also can give patients more time to recover from whatever problem caused the swallowing difficulty. PEG tubes are useful for patients who have trouble swallowing from a variety of chronic neurological impairments (Parkinson's Disease, strokes—brain attack complications) but have good mental function and a quality of life they find acceptable.

There are medical journal articles discussing the safety (low morbidity-illness/mortality) of PEG insertions in the very ill. This safety record seems wonderful. However, what population is getting PEGs? Often it was severely demented elderly. While there is often a discussion on the technical aspects of PEG insertion, whether insertion is an appropriate intervention usually is not mentioned.

Studies have shown that PEG tubes for people with advanced dementia and other severe neurologic impairment did not improve the length or quality of life. Problems with aspiration, decubitus ulcers (bedsores), and muscle wasting still continued. When the length of life was extended, the person was at great risk for painful contractures (permanent muscle tightening) and infection.

If this is the case, why are so many feeding tubes inserted into skilled nursing home residents with advanced dementia? Despite the growing medical literature about the lack of efficacy of feeding tubes in people with advanced dementia, both physicians and families felt otherwise. Regional, religious, gender, and racial differences have been identified. Some areas of the country have more than 50 times the number of PEG tubes inserted than others. Obviously there is more going on in the decision to insert a PEG tube than just medical need.

Many families report being asked by the physician, "You don't want your loved one to starve, do you?" Phrasing the question this way almost demands a certain response. Who is going to reply, "Sure, let him starve." ? The use of the word starving is erroneous. If a person stopped breathing and was not intubated, would that be the equivalent of suffocating them? If a person's kidney's failed and fluid and toxic waste accumulated in their body, would the decision to forego dialysis be the same as drowning or poisoning them?

Feeding someone is a sign of caring and love. Nutrition and nurture come from a single Latin route. As people slip deeper into dementia, their loss of function leads to a more infantile level of functioning. But an infant gets hungry and cries to be fed. The infant's body is geared to take in and utilize the feeding efficiently. The same is not true for the elderly person with advanced dementia. Most of these people are not hungry and are incapable of eating. Most PEG insertions occurred during an admission to an acute care facility for pneumonia, dehydration, and swallowing difficulties. Rather than view these events as part of the dying process, intensive intervention, including acute hospitalization occurred. Fears about aspiration and wishing to avoid complaints weight loss, the institutions may press for the ease of a feeding tube.

People who have voluntarily stopped eating and drinking at the end of their lives report some initial hunger and thirst but little discomfort thereafter. After several days, changes in the body's chemistry lead to a diminished mental capacity as the person slowly loses consciousness. Most of the medical literature supports that death through the lack of oral intake is not uncomfortable, but comfort measures such as mouth care and positioning should be provided.

Sam had a patient who was at the end of his life. He was alert but very frail. Neurological impairment had caused swallowing difficulties but eating remained one of his greatest pleasures. He particularly relished watermelon. The problem was that when he ate, some food would go down the wrong way, and he would cough. To prevent aspiration a feeding tube was inserted. Despite his requests little was given orally. He did not live long with the feeding tube. His family now regrets not giving him the pleasure of eating, especially his watermelon, during the last few weeks of his life.

Proper assistance with meals and comfort feeding can be provided. When the oral intake of a person with advanced dementia declines, various positive steps can be taken without resorting to a feeding tube. Comfort feeding through the relaxation of dietary restrictions and allowing the person to eat whatever they enjoy (food from home) is helpful as is making sure they are rested before meals and positioned correctly. Oral hygiene and properly fitting dentures are critical to insure good intake. Keep the eating environment simple and without distractions is important. Allowing the elder sufficient time to chew and swallow is mandatory.

In some nursing homes and hospitals the staff may not do many simple measures so nutrition becomes compromised. Rushing patients to eat increases the risk for aspiration. We still see patients with food trays lying in bed with their heads barely elevated. Jane once found a patient with a food tray who had both hands in restraints.

Unfortunately, the placement of PEG tubes has almost become a technological imperative—if we can do it we should do it without regard to the appropriateness or outcome. Often in situations where there is little to be done, doing something feels good. It makes us feel as if we are accomplishing something. It nourishes our hope. It also can be a distraction from painful truths. Finally, in the health care system there are rewards for more testing and more treatment and little or nothing (financial or otherwise) for the counseling and support to make the best treatment option.

"I Can't Decide What to Do, So Continue What You are Doing."

Many times a change in health status can come very quickly through a traumatic incident such as a fall or motor vehicle accident, or through a severe acute event such as cardiac arrest or cerebral vascular accident (CVA, stroke or brain attack). For a family member who is faced with making choices in a rapidly shifting situation, decision making is difficult, especially when the diagnosis and prognosis (outcome) is uncertain. Usually the best course of action is to pull out all the stops and do whatever can be done to keep the patient alive until a clearer picture of the pathology and prognosis can be made. This information can be gathered within several days although in some conditions it may take a little longer.

In the best of situations it will be clear that the patient can make a full or good recovery from the current condition and intensive intervention is appropriate and productive. Technological supportive measures such as ventilators, dialysis, and intraortic balloon pumps can be withdrawn as the patient's status improves and the body begins to take over more of its functions independently.

Unfortunately, when the damage is so severe and permanent that the patient will not recover to anywhere near their previous level of functioning.

Some will never regain consciousness. Without the supportive devices the patient would die, but the supportive devices will not improve the underlying pathology or create a better prognosis.

It is very hard for a family to integrate this information when their loved one was fine just a few days before. Sam cared for an elderly woman who had a severe stroke from which she would never recover. In the week before she died, her daughter kept insisting that Sam get a physical therapy consult so her mother could begin rehabilitation.

The families of patients who are experiencing progressive deterioration in health and who have the opportunity (though not all people avail themselves of it) to think about the changes that lie ahead. The families of patients with acute health changes often have given little thought about advanced directives, quality of life issues, or their values related to death and dying. A common response by people in this situation of an acute severe decline in health is to say, "I can't decide what to do, so continue what you're doing." This response allows them to maintain the status quo (assuming that patient's condition does not decline despite intervention) while they process what has happened, gather more information, and make a decision. This is a reasonable position because the choices to be made are critical and should not be rushed into or taken lightly.

However, in some cases this becomes more than a temporary holding position but the default decision making mode. Perhaps emotionally the family members cannot accept the permanent loss of their loved ones as they once were. It could be that the amount of medical information provided is so overwhelming that the family cannot fully process it. Understandably, many people fear making the wrong choice and become paralyzed in their decision making. They would feel tremendously guilty if they make the wrong choice and will probably feel guilty even in making the right choice if the patient's condition does not improve. (See "I Made the Right Choice. Why Don't I Feel Good?) Unclear of what path to take, they stop and fail to move on. Another factor that may impede decision making is the fear of what others may think or do. If they choose to decline more aggressive treatment, the decision to do so may be attacked as being selfish by other family members who are less informed and more in denial.

The hard truth is that there is no way to avoid making difficult decisions. The situation does not allow for it. Even saying, "I can't decide, so continue what you are doing," is a decision—to continue the current treatment plan.

Mrs. Devon was a devoted mother and grandmother who had a major stroke. About a week after the stroke, she still was not responding to the spoken word or even when she was touched. The neurological workup showed that she had suffered severe permanent brain injury. Mrs. Devon was intubated and on a respirator. She had an NG tube for feeding. It was unlikely she would ever be able to breath or eat on her own. This meant she would have to have tubes put into her stomach (PEG tube) and airway (tracheostomy) to keep the tube feedings and ventilation going. The long term prognosis was slow decline from the hazards of immobility (pneumonia, decubitus ulcers--bedsores, and contractures—permanently tightened muscles) and infection.

Mrs. Devon's only child, a son, decided that this was not how she would want to spend the last days of her life and rather than watch her die from the aftermath of her stroke in small steps, he would let the process which had begun a week before continue without intervention. He believed this was the right decision and sadly made his peace with it. However, Mrs. Devon's sister would have none of it. It is likely she did not receive all the information the son had received. Perhaps, the death of her sister was impossible for her to absorb. Perhaps her values and beliefs about life and death were different from her nephew's. In any case, she accused her nephew of killing his mother, of being

142

uncaring, of not wanting to spend the money on her (Medicare would have covered most of the care). It made a very painful situation even more painful. But the son held his position and had her removed from the ventilator. In two days his mother died without any signs of distress. We never learned the outcome of the son's relationship with his aunt.

Removing someone from a ventilator is called weaning. If a person is now capable of breathing independently, the process can be done quite quickly over a few days. If someone has been on a ventilator for a prolonged time, the weaning process may take longer and involve slowly decreasing the level of ventilatory support. People with COPD (chronic obstructive pulmonary disease such as emphysema) who come in for an acute problem such as pneumonia are extremely difficult to wean.

Removing a person from a ventilator who is not expected to breathe independently, terminal weaning, is an entirely different affair. Once the decision has been made and documented, a time is set for the removal of the patient. This allows those who wish to be present the opportunity to be there. The patient's breathing tube is removed and the patient is given low level oxygen through a nasal cannula or face mask. If the patient appears to be in any discomfort, the patient is medicated. Sometimes the patient will stop breathing on their own in a few minutes. Others may linger a day or two. A few, such as in the case of Karen Quinlan who lived for years in a persistent vegetative state, will stabilize and breathe on their own.

Removal of a feeding tube or stopping tube feeding is less dramatic. There is no immediate change. Usually it will take a week to ten days for death to occur. In the meantime the patient should be given good mouth care and kept comfortable. Again how much a person feels at this point is not certain. Most research supports that not providing artificial hydration and nutrition creates an electrolyte disturbance that minimizes discomfort.

Jane cared for an elderly comatose woman, Wilma Revere, who was no longer getting tube feedings because her body was not able to absorb them. The patient was at the very end of life, yet her physician had her IV lines reinserted so she would get hydration and maintain her blood pressure which kept falling. Although her veins were poor and each line lasted only a short while, the doctor kept insisting that another line be started. This continued for two days until she died.

This reinforces the importance of having advanced directives. A living will or health agent could have let Mrs. Revere avoid those unnecessary sticks as she was dying. (See "If I Don't Discuss It, I Won't Die.") Knowing Mrs. Devon's desires should she be in a coma would have given her son more support and may have helped her sister accept his decisions—although sometimes nothing will help.

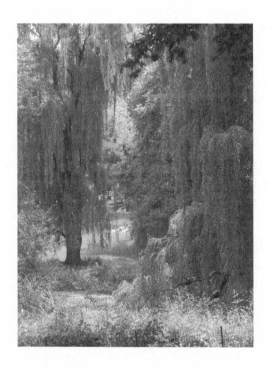

"I Want Everything Done."

Jane works at a community college where part of her service to the college is participating in their speakers' bureau. One of her talks involves keeping emotionally fit as we age and one component of that talk is a discussion of advanced directives. Although Jane always tells people that they should give their health care agent clear guidelines about what they would wish done, she cautions against choosing everything. Her line that "Most people who say they want everything done haven't seen everything," usually gets a laugh but she is very serious about what she is saying. Although this story is not about an older adult, it is such a clear example of the point we want to make that we are including it here.

Jane cared for a man who had AIDS prior to the advances that has allowed it to become more of a chronic disease. In the early 1990's AIDS was a fatal illness that lasted at most a few years. The patient had designated his sister as his health care agent and had told her and written in large print across the health care proxy form, "I want everything done." Certainly part of the patient's fear was being abandoned or given inferior care because of the strong stigma associated with AIDS at this time. He did not want to be ignored. However, in saying and writing what he did, he lost the advantage of having a health care agent—someone who assesses his current health care status and prognosis and makes decisions based on the most accurate information. We do not believe this man envisioned becoming comatose and ventilator dependent. At that point we could no longer discuss treatment options with him. All the invasive lines needed to maintain his life coupled with his depleted immune system led to his body being wracked by one infection after another. A cooling blanket was needed to keep his temperature down. Nothing could be done to reverse the course of his disease. Even comfort measures were limited as the health care providers (HCPs) followed his directive to do everything. His sister was pained by what was happening but felt she had to abide by the patient's wishes. He had a grueling six months of aggressive invasive treatment before he finally succumbed.

The above story is an example of a crisis or a series of crises that were not handled well. The reaction of our society and medical establishment initially to the AIDS epidemic was complicated by discrimination against its earliest victims. This man was in crisis and appeared to have or utilize few resources to help him plan for his care. His sister was left in an untenable position—a health care agent with her hands tied.

Crises are short term situations in which a person's or family's ability to cope with their current stresses becomes overwhelmed. Support systems already in place are insufficient. The chronic illnesses common in the elderly often diminishes their support systems because of their decreased ability to communicate and socialize. People may avoid someone who is sick because they do not know how to respond.

In a crisis, past coping skills—the way we deal with our feelings-- are not helping. Coping skills can be helpful such as praying or talking with a friend or coping skills can be unhealthy such as withdrawing or overeating. Unhealthy coping skills will add to the ongoing crisis.

Coping skills can also be divided into those that deal with release of feelings such as exercise and crying or those coping skills that work to modify the problem situation by learning a new skill and developing new resources. The Chinese character for "crisis" is a combination of the characters for danger and opportunity. A crisis presents the opportunity for growth through the adversity but it also can be a time when maladaptive coping leads to long term dysfunction. Although having a healthy way to deal with feelings is important, if the situation causing the crisis in not addressed, the stress will continue.

Another important factor in dealing with a crisis is having a realistic perception of the situation. When anxiety is high, perception is narrowed and faulty. We may focus on one small aspect of a problem and fail to look at the big picture. We may want something so much that we distort what we see. It is helpful to check assessments of the current situation with others—health care providers, clergy, family, and friends. A word of caution, they may be experiencing their own crisis and may have skewed perceptions of the situation themselves—especially family and friends.

Crises can be caused by one single major event such as receiving a diagnosis of metastatic cancer or it can be an accumulation of smaller events over time. The latter is common in the older adults who have chronic diseases with slower progression of symptoms.

Feeling overwhelmed is a common response to being in a crisis. Physical symptoms include insomnia, fatigue, loss of appetite, and muscle tension. Emotional responses are anxiety, fear, depression, and numbness. In addition, there can be confusion, indecision and poor concentration.

Crises that are the result of health status changes are difficult because just as people are feeling overwhelmed, anxious, and indecisive; they are asked to make some of the most important decisions of their lives. Again this is another reason to have advanced directives in place and to have "the talk" that accompanies them before a crisis occurs. Most people are open to discussions about care options. It is important not to focus on the aspect of withholding and withdrawing treatment, but to discuss choices such as palliative care that could enhance their life, especially toward the end.

Select a time to bring up the discussion about health care agency and end-of-life decision making when there will be few distractions or interruptions. Who broaches the topic first varies. A physician should ask if advanced directives are in place and get specific information about what the patient does or does not desire as far as treatment. Many attorneys create medical advanced directives at the time a will is made. Often the older adult may not remember this. Asking a person if a will exists and then calling the attorney can clarify this and, to some extent, simplify the process.

The older adult may initiate the discussion with a sibling or child who will be the agent or the person who will likely be most involved in the patient's care, may start the discussion to get guidance for the future decision making. When having "the talk," it is important to be specific and honest about the type of care wanted. Play through various scenarios (the physician can be helpful with this) to avoid blanket statements such as, "I never want to be on a ventilator." You may not want to be on a ventilator permanently after a severe head injury, but you may be willing to be on a ventilator for a week while recovering from a chest injury. Discuss your values, goals, and religious beliefs. This will give your agent a better idea of what factors go into your decision making. Ask the agent how they feel about this responsibility and do they feel capable of following your wishes. If possible, give them time to think about it and review the discussion at a later date before completing the simple form. Remember you can always make changes and write a new advanced directive at any time. The one with the most recent date takes priority.

Occasionally when Sam has "the talk" with some of his patients, a few of them will reply, "I don't have anybody." There are people who live very solitary lives or who have outlived their closest contacts. As a health care provider it pays to really press this issue. Very often, when Sam pushes, he finds someone who feels quite close to his patient and health care agency can be established. However if no one can be found, it is important for the person to write a living will outlining much of the same material that was just covered in the discussion on dealing with your agent. Again values, goals, religious beliefs, treatment preferences should be spelt out. A copy should be readily available, perhaps with the physician.

Occasionally, an attorney can both draw up the living will and agree to act as agent. In many cases, if a person has no agent or next of kin, intensive care may be provided that would not have been selected by the person in question.

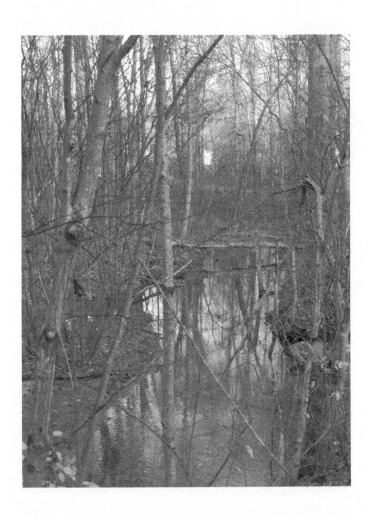

"There Must Be Something Else We Can Do."

Coming to grips with the declining health of a loved one within the limits of the social, environmental, and financial constraints of the situation is never easy. People involved in the decision making often have very different needs and goals. Some may not be able to assess their circumstances realistically because of anxiety, pain, and past emotional history. Time pressures to make decisions add to the stress.

One common response is to delay making a choice as discussed in the section, "I can't decide what to do, so continue what you're doing,." This may appear as if a decision is not being made, but of course it is. Leaving things as they are is a choice and care is given based on that choice. There actually are several advantages to leaving things as they are. The best result is that the problem resolves itself on its own. Although this seems to be more wishful than realistic thinking, it can occur. Sam cared for two people who had cerebral vascular accidents (CVAs, strokes, brain attacks) while at home. Both were already quite debilitated and had expressed the desire not to return to the hospital. With the support of their families, they remained at home. Both survived and regained most of their neurological function without the stress of going through an emergency department and inpatient treatment with all the possibilities for iatrogenic (caused by medical care) injury and illness. These were unique situations and would certainly not apply to most patients with sudden symptoms of a stroke which require immediate treatment to avoid potentially life threatening complications.

Usually leaving things alone in most situations works only temporarily. Typically the loved one's health or the situation deteriorates further and more direct action is forced. The advantage of waiting until this point is that it becomes clearer to (almost) everyone that a change is needed. Trying to get an elderly loved one to use a cane or walker may lead to arguments. However, once someone has fallen and sustained serious injury, deciding about hospitalization and rehabilitation is less likely to cause debate. When decline is obvious, there is less doubt about the need for something to be done and reduced opposition to decisions made in the elder's best interest. This may be to do more, or may be to do less (different).

The downside can be that when intervention comes later and further deterioration has occurred, losses that might have been prevented are now permanent. This may lead to feelings of guilt. Of course, guilt can occur even when the best choices are made and things go as well as they can which is discussed in the section, "I made the right choice. Why don't I feel good about it?"

Often when patients and families refuse to discuss treatment options or make a decision it is because they do not like the options. Life as they have known it has changed irrevocably and circumstances may allow limited choices. Rather than accept this and begin to make reasonable choices within the current situation, the family members spend their time and energy seeking alternatives that do not exist. Sam has seen many people who come to him after they have been to many top specialists for chronic problems and frailty. It is almost as if they think there is a "magic bullet" out there that they are being denied. The acceptance of the fact that there is no "magic bullet" is the first step in seriously considering treatment options that are realistic.

As always there is another side to the story that must be made. Sam had a middle aged patient who brought his mother, an elderly woman with severe COPD (chronic obstructive pulmonary disease), to see Sam because she felt exceedingly weak and tired. The week before his mother was a patient at a major teaching hospital where they ran a battery of tests. It was determined that this woman was at the end of her life and there was nothing more to be done. In desperation, her son brought this frail thin woman to Sam saying, "There must be something else we can do." Sam was dubious that he would have much to offer after the major workup at a medical center. However, he got the woman's records and reviewed them carefully. Sam discovered that the woman had a grossly abnormal thyroid level. The test results had come back after the woman was discharged and no one had looked at them. Treatment for the thyroid condition was straightforward and the elderly woman felt much better.

There are several points to take from this story. One is that even frail elderly people may have some health problems that can be treated and provide significant improvement. Secondly, ask about what tests were done and who reviewed them. There is term, WNL, which usually means "within normal limits." However, some people assume if no one said anything was wrong, then everything is fine. WNL can also mean, "We never looked." Finally, after consultation with several health care experts, delaying decisions about care while trying to get further opinions is not likely to be beneficial. Patients and their loved ones are vulnerable in this situation to quackery which comes in many forms. Be very careful when after consultation with accepted experts in a field someone offers you a solution that seems too good to be true.

"If I Don't Discuss It, I Won't Die."

Neither of us actually ever heard anyone say this but it seems to be an unspoken inner dialogue that guides many people when thinking about advanced directives. There are many misconceptions about the purpose of advanced directives and how they operate which prevents people from creating advanced directives. In New York State decades after putting in place the Health Care Proxy, about a quarter of the population had completed the form. The state recently passed a new law that creates a ranking of who gets to make decisions for the incapacitated adult. We believe advanced directives are crucial in order to provide optimum care not just for the elderly but for all adults. We will address some of these misconceptions that may be preventing you or your loved one from availing yourselves of this important resource.

Some people believe that they do not need an advanced directive because their next of kin will automatically make the decision should they become incapacitated. While this may be true in most cases, the next of kin priority order for the older adult is usually spouse and then children in birth order. We have seen families whose loved one has been estranged from a spouse for decades find out that that spouse is now the health care agent for that loved one. A daughter who provided devoted care to her aged father in her home is displaced as decision maker by an older sibling who has had minimal contact and poor relations with the family for years. If an older adult has no spouse or children, which sibling, cousin, or niece/nephew will assume the role of health care agent? What initially and erroneously seemed like a clear cut issue of who would be the agent can become very complex.

A final thought about just leaving it to whoever is the next of kin—are they capable of the task? Is your spouse or child going to be able to make the hard decisions that may arise or will doing so be too emotionally burdensome? If you are concerned about having your health care wishes carried out, the best thing to do is to select someone who knows what you want and agrees to follow through on you requests. This means you have to talk to your agent prior to appointing them to make your desires known and to assure their acceptance of this important role. It means if you are asked to be an agent that you seek clarification about what that person wants in regard to health care.

The time to do this is now. Advanced directives are not for only those near the end of life. Everyone should have one as we never know what life may bring. It is best done when tensions and emotions are not running high and open discussion can occur. Once someone has had a severe accident, a cerebral vascular accident (CVA, stroke) or is severely demented, it is too late to create an advanced directive.

Your next of kin does not have to be your health care agent. You can appoint anyone except your physician and others who are providing direct patient care. This exclusion is to prevent conflict of interest and delineate the role of decision maker from provider. As mentioned above, you should think carefully about whom you choose as an agent and talk to that person about your concerns. If your agent is not your next of kin, it would be prudent to let your relatives know your choice of agent. This will give you the opportunity to explain your choice and prevent hurt feelings and conflict later.

Some people think that advanced directives are only for people who want to restrict what is done to them (the pull the plug mentality). If they want everything done, they do not need an advance directive. They incorrectly view most health care choices as on-off switches. Either I do something or I do not. A better metaphor would be a rheostat variable resistor such as those used on volume controls or light dimmers. There are levels of choices between on and off.

For the same condition there could be unproven experimental trials, aggressive surgeries, more simple surgical fixes, conservative medical treatment, and watchful waiting. All would have advantages and disadvantages. Some may offer only the smallest chance of recovery. Some may have fewer side effects. The choices are complex and difficult to navigate. Avoiding advanced directives will not insure that everything is done because it is not clear to you or others what "everything" is in many situations. It will make it more likely that your goals and values will not be well addressed

Some people are afraid that if they make an advanced directive they will lose control over their health care decision making. The opposite is the truth. By choosing an agent you can tell someone exactly what are your preferences in health care. You have a greater chance of getting the health care you desire if you are no longer able to speak for yourself. You also eliminate (or at least diminish) the squabbling that often occurs among family about what should be done if you are no longer able to make decisions. The agent cannot interfere with your health care choices as long as you have capacity (able to comprehend benefits, risk, and alternates to treatment) as determined by two physicians. The agent's role only comes into play when it has been determined you are no longer able to make decisions for yourself.

Another misconception about advanced directives is that they are difficult and costly to execute and hard to revise. In fact, they were designed to be very user friendly. Every physician's office, clinic, hospital, nursing home, and rehabilitation center has copies of the advanced directives that comply with their state laws. Many states place blank copies on their health services web sites. However, you do not need an official form. In most states you can write the name of your agent, how to contact them, what directions (if any) you are giving to your agent, and have two witnesses sign the document. In most states it does not need to be notarized. You need to check what form of advanced directives exists where you live.

If you change your mind about who is your agent or what directive you gave, just fill out a new form. The one with the most recent date will take precedence over prior forms. Our suggestion is to either talk to the lawyer that helped prepare your will and have your advanced directives put into place or talk to your physician and have your advanced directive become part of your medical record. Be sure to give your agent a copy and keep a copy handy for yourself.

A healthcare proxy is not the same as a living will. The proxy names a person who will be your agent and will make health care decisions if you lose capacity. This allows for greater responsiveness to your health status. A living will identifies specific treatments and under which circumstances you would either want or not want that care. For example, "If I am ever in a situation where it is felt that the chances of recovering my mental capacity back to its previous state is remote, I do not wish to be kept on a ventilator." One limitation of the living will as an advanced directive is that it is hard to imagine all the possible treatments and circumstances that could occur.

"If I don't discuss it, I won't die," avoids realities and addressing painful feelings and situations. The most important result of creating an advanced directive is often the channels of communication that develop.

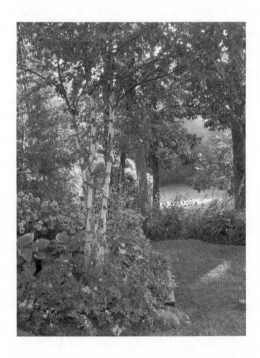

"I Made the Right Choice. Why Don't I Feel Good?"

Many of the situations faced by elderly patients and their families provide limited choices, none of them particularly good. It is emotionally difficult to watch a loved one die slowly poked and prodded by acute care technology, but making the decision to limit or stop treatment is often harder.

The problem is that making a choice cannot be avoided. Allowing everything to be done may be a way of avoiding active decision making and responsibility--doing nothing cognitively or emotionally. But you cannot "do nothing." "Doing nothing" is a choice and leads to certain outcomes. When someone becomes very ill or frail, difficult decisions cannot be escaped.

As discussed in "There Must Be Something Else We Can Do," we would like to find a solution that addresses all our concerns and produces a good outcome. Some people when faced with the dilemma of choosing among less than great treatment options become immobilized and choose nothing—letting the medical establishment run the show. Others will keep asking for and seeking alternatives which is a wonderful thing until alternatives do not exist. Some family members will inflict terrible emotional scars on each other fighting over the right course of action. But one final response to be discussed is when those making the health care treatment choices are realistic, responsible, and caring. They make a choice—whether to limit or withdraw treatment or to utilize every means available to prolong life—after reflecting on the patient's situation, values, and goals.

The problem is that whatever they choose, they still may not feel good about their choice because each outcome still has significant negative consequences. Limiting or withdrawing treatment may reduce the dying process and suffering, but the patient does die sooner. Utilizing every means available to prolong living, still may not achieve that aim, and usually comes at the cost of increased pain and suffering by the patient. Elderly parents may resent the measures taken to keep them safe in their homes, such as home health aides. Others will feel neglected if left alone. Some will feel bitter about placement in a residential facility.

The caregiver/ health care agent trying to do the best he or she can, is usually forced to choose among less than ideal solutions. As there are so many variables that determine what the consequences of any given choice will be, no one can be sure what the outcome will be. The best you can do in this situation is:

- Gather all the information you can
- Get the professionals to tell you their experiences with similar patients.
- Ascertain to the best of your ability what the patient would want and determine if his or her desires are reasonable.

To understand the discomfort behind making difficult end-of-life choices, a background on euthanasia (good death) is needed. Passive euthanasia usually refers to withholding treatments that would likely prolong life. It has two components. One is not providing the treatment in the first place. This would include do not resuscitate (DNR) orders, choosing not to insert feeding tubes, or not placing someone on dialysis or a ventilator. These are usually difficult choices as the patient who requires them is very ill and lacks capacity. The second is removing interventions that have been prolonging life and allowing death to occur naturally. This is often the most uncomfortable option because care is being withdrawn.

Although most moral theorists do not see a difference between these two forms of passive euthanasia, some religions do. And for most people, psychologically it is easier not to have started something than to stop it. Again, we want to reiterate, when a person has a sudden change in health status and the prognosis is unclear, it is worthwhile to employ aggressive measures to maintain life while the situation is assessed. If the prognosis comes back that permanent severe damage has occurred, the agent or family, guided by their understanding of the patient's wishes may be doing the best thing by discontinuing treatment.

Active euthanasia is performing an action that will cause the patient's death, such as administering an overdose. (This is different than giving the patient sufficient medication to manage pain even though it might impair respirations. The goal in this case is to decrease pain, not stop respirations). Active euthanasia, also called mercy killing, is illegal in this country and forbidden by health care professional codes of conduct.

Physician assisted suicide (PAS) is legal in two states, Oregon and Washington. In PAS the physician provides the patient with the medication to take that will comfortably stop the patient from breathing and induce death. This is done only after strict criteria have been met. We have not had any experience with PAS, but have cared for people who requested it. The idea of having control over their dying process (whether they would have used PAS or not) was comforting to these people.

When faced with having to select from among limited options with significant downsides, the older adult, caregivers, and health care agents soon learn that choice does not equal feeling good about what we must decide. Choice does not equal control.

Some concluding thoughts about end of life decision making. We have emphasized the importance of having good communication among the elderly, their families, and their health care providers. The first step is to assist older adults in clarifying their needs, goals, desires, and fears. Creating a quiet, unrushed, nonjudgmental environment for this dialogue is essential. This is an ongoing process as situations change and is unlikely to be accomplished in one session. Secondly, in choosing a health care agent, the elder must consider the potential agent's ability to carry out the elder's wishes and live with the consequences. This recognizes that making and living with difficult health care choices among less than ideal options is emotionally draining for the agent. If you feel the person closest to you would be overly burdened by this responsibility, explain your reasons behind choosing another agent as coming from a caring place not as rejection. Finally, although agents may not feel good about the decisions and their outcomes, agents may feel a sense of accomplishment in fulfilling the responsibility entrusted to them.

Section Five: Beyond the Stories—
Thoughts to Consider

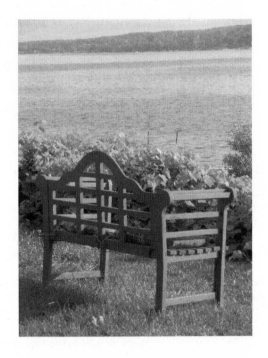

The Serenity Prayer

God grant me the serenity
To accept the things I cannot change;
Courage to change the things I can;
And wisdom to know the difference.

Reinhold Niebuhr

Futile Care and Health Care Decision Making

Our goal is to find the most compassionate respectful care that has the greatest authenticity to the person receiving the care. Our goal at the end of life with the elderly, becomes directed at preserving the quality of life as much as possible rather than extending life at any cost. Understanding the concepts of futile care and health care decision making is important in achieving these goals.

The term, futile care, is difficult to define. In general, it is care that is unlikely to provide any benefit to the patient. More specifically, medical futility can be defined as care that fails to prolong life significantly or to improve the quality of life. Our health care system is continually developing new interventional technologies and medications which is a wonderful thing. One by-product, however, is that people are living longer but sicker and often experiencing prolonged periods of painful dying. Providing futile care at this time in the course of the illness will do no good but will increase the period of suffering. "Doing everything" may seem like the loving moral thing to do, but it can also be a refuge for those who do not really want to examine a painful situation or for those who lack the emotional strength to say "no" to the death denying juggernaut of high tech care. This requires stopping the natural reflex to respond to every health problem with another possible, if unlikely, fix.

Deciding what is futile care is not an exact science. There are many variables to consider which in some situations make the determination of futility difficult. Other times it is quite obvious to those who pause and look at the big picture. Before reacting to each new health crisis with some new intervention, there is the opportunity to consider the patient's current status and realistic prognosis. Yet for many health care providers and family members, there is no such thing as futile care. It is an issue they never want to address because it shows the limited abilities of health care providers and acceptance of the mortality of the loved one.

When health care is viewed through the acute care lens under the misguided perspective that such treatment will rectify illnesses and restore the patients to their previous health, every possible treatment option must be performed. This outlook shows little regard to the fact that there may be insurmountable underlying chronic and progressive illnesses, the extreme loss of functioning seen in the frail elderly, or such significant permanent changes from the previous health status to render acute care impotent. It is not a question of treating this complication and then that complication, but looking at what is the patient's overall health status and prognosis.

What are the downsides to futile care? The most important downside to futile care is putting the patient through the unnecessary discomfort and pain that often accompanies additional useless tests and treatments. Even a common simple procedure such as drawing blood for lab tests can be difficult and painful when a patient has poor veins or generalized edema (swelling). Recent studies have shown that some hospitalized patients actually acquire anemia from having their blood drawn so frequently. Will the test provide any useful additional information or are the tests being done because of some protocol? The ethical discussion on futility focuses on the balance between nonmaleficence (do no harm) and beneficence (do good). When a test or treatment will not help the patient then exposing the patient to the complications that may arise is wrong. Futile treatment should not be offered because all treatments have risks and if there is no good achieved for the patient who should at least be protected from unnecessary risk.

Another downside is that the continual pursuit of health in the acute care mode delays looking at palliative measures that can truly improve the patient's quality of life by addressing comfort issues. When patients are more comfortable, they sleep and eat more which may actually extend life. They will be less delirious and be able to cooperate more in their care rather than needing restraints or sedation. They can participate more in decision making. The continual pursuit of acute care mode usually delays everyone from looking at the overall trend in the patient's health. Futile care can distract patients and their families from having important end of life discussions.

When the patient is unable to participate in decision making, the family then is asked to make decisions. We have heard health care providers say that they know they are administering futile treatments but they are doing so because it makes the family feel better. (This is different than allowing time to thoroughly assess the situation before deciding on care.) We should not be treating patients to make their family members feel better. This shows a lack of respect for the patients who now are treated not based on their needs, but on those of the family. We have elevated the maintenance of their bodies at the expense of their personhood.

Discussing financial consideration of end of life often makes people uncomfortable. A meaningful discussion of futile care which includes its financial cost can be hijacked by emotional terms such as "death panels" or "rationing." Yet spending huge amount of health care dollars on treatments that accomplish little for the patient's welfare (or even harms the patient) would seem to be clearly wrong. The idea of medical futility needs to be addressed by our society. Currently we are paying huge amounts of money for very little gain. About 12% of all Medicare payments come during the last month of life. Most of this cost is providing acute care to patients with terminal or end stage chronic illnesses for which the treatment was never originally intended. As a society, we seem willing to spend tremendous amounts of money for futile intensive care at the end of life while under funding measures such as home health aides and senior rides which would accomplish more for the quality of life for a larger elderly population. Better provision of basic needs for food and supervision in homes and residences would probably reduce hospitalizations and the downward spiral that occurs as people get frail with age.

In the discussion on health care ethics (in the next chapter of Section Five) the principles of justice and utility will be presented in more depth. Briefly, the principle of justice demands a fair distribution of resources. The principle of utility emphasizes do the greatest good for the greatest number. Spending large amounts of money on marginally useful treatment at the end of a person's life when preventative health measures are underfunded would be in conflict with these two ethical guidelines.

Studies have shown that many health care providers (HCP) have delivered care to terminally ill patients and the elderly at the end of their lives that the HCPs found morally disturbing. Although some cases deal with under-treatment during this stage of life, the vast majority of cases are instances of overtreatment that extended the dying process and the patients' suffering. The HCPs had difficulty determining between what was an extraordinary measure (such as mechanical ventilation) and what was an ordinary measure (such as the provision of hygiene) and how best to respect a patient's values.

Cardiopulmonary Resuscitation (CPR) is an example of a very valuable intervention that at times is futile and should be withheld. As in most treatment options, the issue is not whether CPR is an extraordinary or ordinary measure but rather its appropriateness in certain clinical situations. CPR was originally developed and intended for use in acute reversible cardiac arrest. The population intended to be served by this intervention were patients without progressive terminal illnesses or severely debilitating chronic illnesses, but the cardiac patient (or choking or near drowning patient) with a dysrhythmia (abnormal electrical activity in the heart) who would respond to straightforward treatment and regain a significant quality of life. There was an expansion of the use of CPR to larger and larger populations whose need for such treatment is not as clear and who would in many cases receive much less benefit from this intervention. Various studies have shown survival rates for Medicare patients who receive CPR in the hospital are at best 20% and most report much lower levels of success. That is, at best only 1 in 5 elders who receive

CPR in the hospital get discharged. Those who did survive tended to have been admitted with much better baseline health levels and fewer underlying chronic health problems. The quality of life and the recuperation to previous health levels for those who were discharged after receiving CPR are rarely discussed.

The cessation of cardiac activity is part of everyone's dying process. The reluctance to separate out the intended population for CPR from all dying patients has led to the expectation that all patients would receive CPR unless Do Not Resuscitate (DNR) orders were given. Although this initially may seem generous and humane--doing all one can--it is actually mindless and fails to individualize care to what the patient needs. The technological imperative -- if we can do it, we do it, no questions asked--has taken over reasoning.

Perhaps technological hubris would be a better term. If I am capable of doing something whether it will help or not, then I must do it. This approach almost eliminates the need for reflection and critical thinking—a one size (ventilator, PEG tube, dialysis, and blood pressure medications) fits all mentality. It takes a lot more time and interpersonal contact to explain to a family why "doing everything" may not be the best choice for their loved one. It is easier to just order more tests and treatments. It is simpler for the HCP to start by providing the patient and family a list of all the treatment options (not always including palliative measures) than to clarify the patient's health status, prognosis, and goals. Therefore, doing everything often is the easiest approach.

The advice by health care providers to do more may have other motivations than the patients' best interests. Some providers may want the opportunity to perform a new technique or use some new equipment. Other reasons for suggesting more treatment may be to provide opportunities to teach students, to conduct research, or provide patients for specific programs such as hyperbaric treatment or open heart surgery. These are not necessarily bad goals, but it is a problem if those making the decision about patient care (patients and family) have no idea that there are other motives other than their loved ones' welfare affecting the advice they are given.

Patients and their families may wish for everything to be done, including CPR, because they fear abandonment by health care professionals. Asking for everything to be done may seem the way to show their own concern for the patient. They may view the opposite of doing everything as doing less which sounds uncaring. Reframing the discussion from doing less to doing different may help. Pushing harder with acute care may bring less benefit to the patient than switching to a less aggressive, palliative mode.   There is a need to explore all treatment options--focusing on what best serves the patient at this time without labeling the interventions as "more" or "less" care.

Making these deeply personal and difficult decisions is compounded by the complexity of the situation.   The language, the technology, and the unfamiliarity   of   the   environment   can   be overwhelming to patients and families who are tired and in pain. We hope this area of aggressive futile intervention will be resolved in the next few years. But with new technologies and interventions being developed all the time, this may be an unrealistic goal.

Ethical Reasoning

The method for deliberating about ethical issues is both logical and compassionate at the same time. The combination of reason and feeling provides against the extremes of responding only based on our feelings or cold logic. We want to balance both. Ethical decisions are not just doing what feels right. Nor are ethical decisions abstract impersonal calculations that rationalize away the core of humanity. Adherence only to ethical principles in a rote fashion would fail to address the complexity and uniqueness of real life situations. Gut feelings are important but hard to communicate to others. Intellect must be brought to the process.

When trying to make decisions about what type and level of health care to give, family and health care providers will look to ethics as one source of guidance. Ethics is a field of philosophy that deals with the rightness or wrongness of actions. Bioethics is a subdivision of ethics that deals with health care. Health care is closely linked to ethics because it evokes questions about basic human values. Patients, families, and health care providers (HCPs) are participants in the most personal, traumatic, wonderful, and painful experiences in our lives.

The five moral principles that have grounded health care are:

1. nonmaleficence--do no harm
2. beneficence--do good
3. autonomy--respect for individuals
4. justice--fair allocation of costs and benefits of health care
5. utility--using health care resources where they will do the greatest good for the greatest number.

Certain courses of action may support one principle while defying another. For example, we readily accept that to do good we often bring some harm or risk of harm to the patient. Necessary surgery causes pain, scarring, and the potential for infection. Antibiotics can cause nerve and renal damage.

In respecting a patient's autonomous desire to have "everything" done in their care, we may violate the principles of nonmaleficence, justice, and utility. Inappropriate care exposes patients to health care related risks with little or no benefit. Unnecessary care stands in opposition to the principle of utility and perhaps justice when huge amounts of money are spent to extend lives a few more days or weeks.

These five principles create patient rights which in turn create duties in those who care for them. Some of these are negative duties--do no harm. This means avoid doing something bad or wrong. For

179

example operating on the wrong side of the body would clearly be doing harm. Other actions may be more difficult to define as harmful or not. Many therapeutic medications and treatments such as chemotherapy and radiation have significant and serious side effects.

Some of duties are positive--do good. Maintaining confidentiality is an example of doing good. But in the case where someone with a mental illness poses a clear threat to themselves or another person confidentiality must be waived.

How good is good enough? Most bioethical systems draw a line between ordinary measures of care which must be given (and in some cases cannot even be refused) and extraordinary measures that may not be offered to everyone and can be refused. For example, a person cannot say they do not believe in the germ theory and ask a surgeon not to use sterile technique. That is considered ordinary care. On the other hand, the same person could decline blood products, dialysis, and a pacemaker which are considered extraordinary measures.

When determining whether an intervention would be categorized as ordinary or extraordinary, it is most important to look at the big picture for this particular person. What are his or her goals and values? How will the intervention impact the prognosis and quality of life? What is the purpose of

180

the treatment? Will it enhance the person's life or just prolong an uncomfortable dying process?

For example, DNR—do not resuscitate, DNI—do not intubate, and AND—allow natural death are examples of orders to limit extraordinary interventions. The decision is made either by a patient with capacity (able to know the risks, benefits, and alternatives to treatment) or the patient's health care agent. The physicians and staff caring for the patient may have their own personal perspectives on whether these orders are appropriate. Some may feel that DNR orders are never appropriate. Others health care providers may feel uncomfortable raising the topic to the patient and family. Still others may feel frustrated and sad resuscitating a patient they believe will never be saved.

Ethical dilemmas and conflicts arise when guidelines established by the moral community fail to provide a definitive answer to the questions raised in a particular situation. Dilemmas tend to cluster around new technology and changing social ideals. The community as a whole works through philosophical and legal cases to build a consensus which clarifies and gives expanded guidelines for practice. One area where this can be seen in process but not resolved is the placement and removal of artificial feeding devices for patients in irreversible comas.

The principle of autonomy offers a way to negotiate some of these conflicts by requiring the patient/family to give informed consent to invasive procedures. But often this consent is requested at times of extreme emotional distress or the information provided does not lay the foundation for real understanding and choice for the patient and agent.

There are many forces that have impacted on the health care system and increased the likelihood of ethical concerns. They are:

1. The aging population of patients--who have more complex and long term health care needs.

2. An increase in the severity of illness among patients. Patients who in the recent past would have been hospitalized are now receiving home care. Those who in the hospital would have been in ICU's are now on the general floors. And the level of care demanded of ICU patients continues to escalate.

3. The development of advanced technology and more invasive monitoring and treatment techniques that has on one hand allowed us to maintain patients who would have previously died, but at the

cost of a diminishing of quality of life due to pain, immobility, and loss of privacy.

4. Patient and their families arriving at the hospital during emergency situations, with little or no preparation. The technical language, the space age machinery, and the complicated care are hard for them to comprehend, especially with the added stressors of high anxiety and physical illness.

5. Patients and their families responding to these invasive technologies and perceived threats to the quality of life by demanding increased respect for their autonomy resulting in emphasis on issues such as informed consent and surrogate decision making for incapacitated patients.

6. Finally, to further add complexity to the system, there is the pressure to increase efficiency and cost effectiveness. A variety of governmental, business, and consumer groups are expecting the health care provider to deliver the most sophisticated, individualized care to the sickest of patients and to be thrifty too! As we change the semantics of those for whom we care from patients, to clients, to health care consumers, what are we saying about our perception of

the relationship and the responsibilities that exist between the care giver and care receiver?

Most health institutions have ethics committees in place, They have broad membership — physicians, nurses, social workers, pharmacists, chaplains, lawyers, and community representatives. The ethics committee helps set policy for the hospital and provides education on bioethical matters. Patients and their families can request a consult from the ethics committee when they believe their rights have not been properly respected or when there is conflict about treatment options. The decisions of the ethics committee are usually not binding but in some cases they may limit the treatment options available.

Here are some suggestions to help think about the ethical implications of health care decisions.

1. Identify who should be involved in decision making.

   Is everyone who should be included part of the process? Is anyone who should not be included involved? Resentments by staff, patients, and families often result from the exclusion from the process no matter what decision is reached. Conflicts arise when those who should be involved in the process have not been included. This can lead to confusion about how decisions were made. Of course, involvement of more people increases likelihood of divergent opinions. Advanced directives were made part of our legal system to clarify who gets to make decisions when the patient becomes incapacitated, but discussing the situation and options with others may make them accept the decision more readily.

2. Gather as much pertinent information as possible about the situation and where possible get agreement on the facts of the situation.

The more information available the better the decision usually will be and the more confidence there will be in the choice. For example, if family and friends can supply past comments made by the patient about quality of life and end of life care, choices of treatment for a comatose patient can be more reflective of the patient's values

Agreement on the facts is critical. If not all people believe the patient is in a persistent vegetative state (permanent loss of all higher brain functioning), then it is unlikely that they will support the same course of action. If consensus is not reached, see if further information may help. Sometimes additional information will not help because of an inability to handle a painful truth. If the refusal to face facts is more a result of the emotional defense of denial, then pastoral and emotional support may be of some use. This is the occasion for gently providing realistic perspectives on the situation. When possible, a little time for family members to adjust to terrible situations can help.

3. Identify and prioritize key issues or problems.

Anticipating future needs and potential problems will help prevent small issues from magnifying into major conflicts. It is also very important to realize that all potential solutions will have both positive and negative aspects. Rarely will an option present itself without a downside. Those who have expectations of a perfect solution can obstruct positive reasonable actions while chasing a non-attainable ideal. Therefore it is essential to be realistic about solutions and help all involved accept legal, financial, and other real life limitations. It means that expectations should not be set so high that nothing that can actually be done is acceptable.

Many issues that at first seem like major ethical issues actually turn out to be legal, psychological, or some other type of problem. Once correctly identified as to its key area, interventions are more likely to be efficient and successful. Not everyone may agree on every point but there should be some areas of agreement where work can begin. Help can than be requested from specific people such as social workers or occupational therapists to deal with particular problems. Also consultation with a health agency's ethics committee can be of value. It some rare cases where there is great conflict, it may be mandatory.

4. Show empathy for the feelings of others involved in the situation

Each person has his or her own perspective, relationship with the patient and interpretation of the events. Taking time to explore the sources of the each person's feelings is important. Identifying and acknowledging other people's perspectives will decrease the development of conflict. This does not mean one has to agree with or accept another's point of view, but all should be treated respectfully.

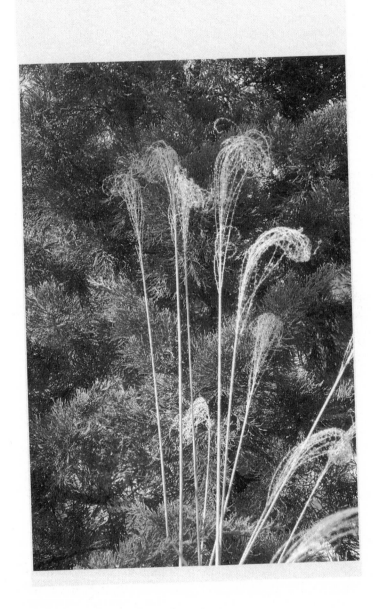

Levels of Dementia (see pp. 35-36)

Area of Function	Mild	Moderate	Severe
Cognitive (Mental) Capabilities Memory, Orientation, Executive Function (problem solving and organizational skills, judgment)	Moderate loss of recent memory beginning to impact functioning Difficulties with time and place orientation Difficulties with problem solving and impaired judgment	Severe memory loss; difficulty learning new information Significantly disoriented to time and place Executive Function significantly diminished Social interaction impaired	Severe memory loss including short and long term memory Oriented to person but may not recognize self in mirror Lacks judgment and ability to problem solve
Activities of Daily Living (ADL's) hygiene, dressing, toileting, eating, mobility	Performance of self-care is diminished and not recognized	Needs assistance with self-care	Needs great assistance with self-care; Incontinence
Instrumental Activities of Daily Living (IADL's) cooking, shopping, managing finances, housekeeping	Impairment in ability to perform skills related to household maintenance	Can perform only simple household tasks	Unable to contribute to the functioning of the household

A Prayer for Healing

Hope in God; Be strong and let your heart take courage; Hope in God.   (Psalms 27:14)

Merciful God, we pray to you for the recovery of _____. O God, let each of these persons experience a complete recovery-- a healing of body, mind, and spirit. Grant each of our loved ones renewed strength and confidence. Give wisdom and skill to those who help in healing. Help all of us who share the anxiety of these illnesses, injuries, and infirmities to be brave, cheerful, and hopeful.

O God, we pray for all those in our hearts to be speedily healed, but we know that some may be near their life's end, if this is so, we pray that You grant them a gentle death and let them pass with grace knowing that their lives have touched others for good and been filled with meaning.

Merciful One, inspire us with courage and faith. Grant your blessings for healing to those who call upon You. O God, who blessed our fathers, Abraham, Isaac, and Jacob, and mothers, Sara, Rebecca, Rachel, and Leah, send your blessings to _____. Have mercy on them, and graciously restore them to health and strength. Grant them a complete recovery, a healing of spirit, and a healing body, along with all who are stricken in Israel. May healing come speedily, and let us say: Amen.

By Rabbi Marc Gruber

Made in the USA
Middletown, DE
11 February 2017